"Zoltán Dörnyei is one of the most formidable researchers I know. In this characteristically fascinating book he traverses a number of usually distinct intellectual worlds to offer us an account of vision which is rich, inspiring and also practical. I can think of no one else who could bring together neuroscience, social science, business and theology into a work so useful and interesting as this one."

– **Karen Kilby**, Bede Professor of Catholic Theology, Durham University, UK

"In this book, Zoltán Dörnyei offers a masterful multifaceted exploration of vision through the prism of his cross-disciplinary expertise in science and theology. Substantial, insightful, and practice-oriented, this seminal work is essential reading for anyone wanting to more fully understand and experience the power of vision in Christian life and ministry."

– **Carolyn Kristjánsson**, PhD, CEC, Trinity Western University, Canada

"We are living in times when many people, both individually and collectively, are seeking purpose in their lives and are longing to discern a vision for a more hopeful future. By bringing together two distinctive lines of inquiry across the social sciences and theology, this book represents a new kind of scholarship, one that reaches imaginatively across these disciplines while at the same time offering concrete practical proposals to any community compelled to respond to vision in action."

– **Maggie Kubanyiova**, Professor of Language Education, University of Leeds, UK

Vision, Mental Imagery and the Christian Life

This book uniquely explores how the notion of vision is presented in modern science and the Bible, and how it can be applied to contemporary Christian contexts. The word "vision," our ability to see, has been described by an increasing body of scholarship in the social sciences as our capacity for mental imagery and imagination. As such, this unique cognitive capability has been utilised in many fields for a variety of purposes, from arts and psychotherapy to politics and business management, and even for performance enhancement in sports.

The current book argues that a better understanding of vision can have far-reaching practical implications for Christian life and ministry by helping people to align themselves with God's specific purposes. After a theoretical overview that integrates scientific and theological insights, the final chapters present a variety of strategies that can help believers to discern God's call through the use of mental imagery and then to develop and cultivate the perceived vision.

The book examines the scientific and biblical principles of vision in a comprehensive manner, with a special emphasis on the practical implications of the issue. As such, it will be of great interest to scholars of Theology, Biblical Studies and Church Growth/Leadership, as well as Organisational Behaviour, Business Management and Psychology.

Zoltán Dörnyei is Professor of Psycholinguistics in the School of English, University of Nottingham (UK). During the past three decades he has published over 100 academic papers and 25 books on various aspects of the psychology of second language acquisition. Parallel to his main job, Zoltán has also undertaken training in theology: he obtained an MA in biblical interpretation and a second PhD in Theology at Durham University (UK). His publications in this area include *Christian Faith and English Language Teaching and Learning* (2013, New York: Routledge; with M. Wong and C. Kristjánsson) and *Progressive Creation and the Struggles of Humanity in the Bible: A Canonical Narrative Interpretation* (2018, Eugene, OR: Pickwick).

Routledge New Critical Thinking in Religion, Theology and Biblical Studies

The *Routledge New Critical Thinking in Religion, Theology and Biblical Studies* series brings high quality research monograph publishing back into focus for authors, international libraries, and student, academic and research readers. This open-ended monograph series presents cutting-edge research from both established and new authors in the field. With specialist focus yet clear contextual presentation of contemporary research, books in the series take research into important new directions and open the field to new critical debate within the discipline, in areas of related study, and in key areas for contemporary society.

For more information about this series, please visit: www.routledge.com/religion/series/RCRITREL

Vision, Mental Imagery and the Christian Life

Insights from Science and Scripture

Zoltán Dörnyei

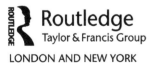
Routledge
Taylor & Francis Group

LONDON AND NEW YORK

First published 2020 by Routledge

2 Park Square, Milton Park, Abingdon, Oxon, OX14 4RN
605 Third Avenue, New York, NY 10017

Routledge is an imprint of the Taylor & Francis Group, an informa business

First issued in paperback 2020

Copyright © 2020 Zoltán Dörnyei

British Library Cataloguing-in-Publication Data
A catalogue record for this book is available from the British Library

Library of Congress Cataloging-in-Publication Data
A catalog record for this book has been requested

ISBN: 978-1-138-47833-6 (hbk)
ISBN: 978-0-367-78580-2 (pbk)

Typeset in Sabon
by Apex CoVantage, LLC

Contents

Foreword

Walt Disney died while the Disney World Theme Park in Florida was under construction. At its opening in 1971, an official is said to have commented to his widow, "What a pity Walt Disney didn't live to see this day." "Oh," she replied, "but he did see it." He may have died before it was completed but he had a vision, a vision that led him to build the "Magic Kingdom" and EPCOT (the Experimental Prototype Community of Tomorrow) in the first place. Vision is a powerful motivating factor, leading us to see a different world and release unrealised potential.

Vision, though, is a spacious word, which is defined differently and used variously in a wide range of fields. It most obviously refers to external physical stimuli which we see with our eyes. But it also relates to receiving inner stimuli which can be just as real and powerful, to a vision for the future as beloved by business people, to a mental image of victory which motivates sports competitors. It also occurs greatly in the Bible to describe the experience of the people of God. The Old Testament prophets had their visions, some described in spectacular and memorable detail, while Peter announced the democratisation of that gift on the Day of Pentecost. From then on, he said, Joel's prophecy would be fulfilled and many, young and old alike, would have visions and dreams as a sign of living in the last chapter of earth's history. Paul speaks of the vision he had, while John records one long and often mysterious vision which becomes the climax of Scripture in the book of Revelation. What, if anything, do these different uses of vision have in common, or are they entirely different, unrelated, experiences? It is here that Zoltán Dörnyei's skills as a respected social scientist, qualified theologian and gifted teacher come into play.

This book achieves a number of things which are highly unusual and, in some cases, even unique. First, it maps the importance of vision in Scripture and Christian experience. As an evangelical shaped by the Reformation, my emphasis has been on words. I have never dismissed visions, especially the Biblical ones, but neither have I really had a place for them or known quite what to do with them. Zoltán has opened my eyes to their importance in Scripture and led me to new understandings and an enriched balance of the complementarity of what is seen as well as heard.

Second, the book uses contemporary social science and its understanding of vision and motivation to portray the subject on a wide canvas and explain what is happening when people have a vision. Social science is used not to reduce or undermine Christian experience, as crude social science has sometimes illegitimately done, but to illuminate it. As an accomplished teacher, Zoltán is able to explain complex social science research in a very accessible form, without over-simplifying it, and apply it to our contemporary experience and lives.

Third, therefore, the book serves as a model of integration between Scripture and social science. It is like the end of a television detective drama where all the pieces fall into place and we say, "Ah, that's what was going on!" We certainly need to be discerning rather than naïve in our use of the social sciences, but since "all truth is God's truth," we have a lot to learn from contemporary research. It is to be hoped that others will use this book as a model of integration which they imitate in their own field and writing. As one who studied sociology in the 1960s, I only wish such an example of integrating the two different fields of sociology and theology had been available then.

Fourth, the book helps to explain the shift of emphasis in the church between vision as an in-breaking, "supernatural" event – a revelation from beyond – and vision as having a dream about what the church should aim to look like in the future, which has contributed to the formation of many a mission statement. The motivational power of vision in business and sports is particularly relevant here.

Fifth, the book is full both of biblical faithfulness and pastoral wisdom. As a committed charismatic, Zoltán is very familiar with the gift of vision as experienced in charismatic churches and not sceptical about them. But neither is he unaware of associated problems. In several chapters he sets out practical and godly wisdom for discerning what visions are authentic and how to handle them and the over-enthusiasm of some who misuse them.

As mentioned in passing earlier, this book is like a good detective series on the TV. When my wife and I begin to watch one, we often comment on how many stories and people are in play at the start and how we are struggling to see how they are related to each other or the main story line. As the episodes unfold, we begin to see connections we had missed until in the end it all falls into place and makes sense. Clarity replaces confusion. That's what happens here as Zoltán Dörnyei uses his training and experience to explore the theme of vision from several angles.

Within the church, the subject of vision, or visions, has been a controversial issue for many years. Some enthusiastically embrace them as a sign of the Holy Spirit at work without exercising any thought or discernment about them. At the other end of the spectrum, there are others who dismiss them wholesale as belonging to a different age and as having been rendered redundant by the completion of the canon of Scripture. In between, there are some who see their value in other cultures, since they cannot deny the number of, say, Muslims who are converted to Christ by having a vision rather than by hearing a human preacher, but who do not entertain them in western culture. Still others are happy with the more "secularised" understanding of vision as when we use it to speak of a "vision statement," whether in business or church, but are uneasy about what charismatic friends understand by a vision.

Zoltán Dörnyei's book has something to offer and to challenge all, wherever we fall in the kaleidoscope of positions about vision. I hope it is widely read and studied, since it will enrich both our personal discipleship and the church's experience of God, and in some measure help us to understand one another, therefore promoting the peace which the Holy Spirit gives.

– Derek Tidball, Former Principal of the London
School of Theology and former
Chairman of the Evangelical Alliance, UK

Acknowledgements

It was Pastor Nick Sharp who first highlighted to me the possible Christian applications of my scientific research on vision – thank you for your encouragement! I am also grateful to several friends – Carolyn Kristjansson, Jon Potter, Ben Topliss and Mary Shepard Wong – for their generous support at various stages of preparing the manuscript. I am particularly thankful to Derek Tidball for all his thoughtful comments, which have shaped the material right from the beginning, as well as for writing the kind Foreword. Finally, I owe a debt of gratitude to my wife, Sarah, who has helped me in so many ways, including offering detailed suggestions on many aspects of the text.

Copyright

Introduction

The nature and significance of vision

In the English language, the word "vision" is commonly used both in everyday parlance and in a variety of professional contexts, and it is a term that most people can readily relate to, even beyond its core meaning of "eyesight." This is a reflection of the widespread belief that the term has profound relevance to a broad spectrum of human experiences and affairs. Indeed, the notion of vision has been employed widely in a number of different domains, from politics and psychotherapy to business management and anthropology. In our current age, not only does every prominent politician and company CEO purport to have a vision, but so do many human rights campaigners, artists and educators to name a few, and the spectrum of individual visions is further complemented by manifold examples of institutional vision held by, for example, universities, commercial enterprises, community centres and even ballet companies! Vision has also been an important theological concept due to frequent occurrences of the term in the Scriptures, each carrying significant meaning – some would go as far as to say that the Bible itself is largely a product of visionary experiences. Over the past three decades the term has also emerged as a dominant theme in the Christian literature on church growth and church leadership, often seen as a decisive factor concerning the state of the contemporary church in the west.

Thus, in an insightful review article, Ruud van der Helm rightly concludes that "visions show up in diverse contexts, taking many different shapes,"[1] so much so that we can talk about "the vision phenomenon" to cover "the ensemble of claims and products which are called 'visions' or could be called as such."[2] Yet, despite this relatively high profile, there have been surprisingly few focused treatises written on vision in biblical scholarship, and even in the social sciences we find a great deal of misunderstanding, superficial interpretation and somewhat contradictory conceptualisation surrounding the term. It is therefore useful to begin the exploration of the topic with an introductory chapter that lays the foundations for the subsequent discussion

---

1 van der Helm, "The Vision Phenomenon," 96.
2 Ibid.

by examining the exact nature and significance of vision. After an initial stocktaking of the multiple meanings that the term covers, we will move on to address four pertinent issues: the benefits of integrating scientific and theological insights in understanding the nature of vision; the significance of the notion of vision in both fields; the difference between vision and other related concepts (e.g. imagination and revelation); and finally, possible ways in which vision can enrich Christian life and ministry. The Introduction will conclude with suggestions on how to read the material selectively if time is at a premium.

The meaning of the term "vision"

Even the most cursory exploration of the term "vision" reveals that it has several different meanings. In contemporary English, the word occurs in at least three distinct senses:

(a) *Physical perception*, which is commonly used to refer to someone's eyesight, for example in sentences such as "*My vision has deteriorated since last time*" or "*Pilots need perfect vision.*"
(b) *Mental picture*, which concerns various forms of internal images and visualisations such as memory images, daydreams, fantasies, creative imagination and spiritual revelations (e.g. prophetic image). This "internal sight" has been captured expressively in the phrase "mind's eye," as coined by Shakespeare in a dialogue from his play *Hamlet*, where the title character explains: "*My father – methinks I see my father. / Where, my lord? / In my mind's eye, Horatio.*"[3]
(c) *Future aspiration*, which is a meaning frequently ascribed to the ambitions of politicians or business leaders in contexts such as "*Walt Disney's vision was to establish a theme park in California.*"

Thus, in the English language "vision" can refer either to seeing something through one's *physical eyes* or in the *mind's eye*, and in the latter case it can also denote *foreseeing* a picture of a desired future in one's imagination.[4] In the *British National Corpus*, which is a digitalised, 100-million-word collection of samples of written and spoken language from a wide range of sources,[5] we find more than 4,000 occurrences of the word, mostly

---

3 Act 1, Scene 2. Although Shakespeare is usually credited with coining the term, a version of the phrase also appears in the Man of Law's Tale in Chaucer's *Canterbury Tales* (end of 14th century), where we read about a blind Christian man who could only see with the "eyes of his mind" ("*eyen of his mynde*").
4 We should note, however, that although these three different meanings are expressed by the same word in English, this is not necessarily the case in other languages; in Hungarian, for example, we find a different word for each semantic referent.
5 See www.natcorp.ox.ac.uk/.

corresponding to these three semantic domains; interestingly, however, the meaning that most people would probably judge to be the basic reference of the term, physical perception, is in fact only the second most common usage. The most popular meaning of vision concerns the third option listed earlier, that is, a hoped-for, desirable future state or plan. This meaning has become particularly popular in business and political discourse over the past four decades to refer to the envisaged future goals and mission plans of prominent leaders or successful companies (e.g. "*Mr. A's predecessor had the vision of a large, permanent staff . . .*"), but the *British National Corpus* confirms that the term also occurs widely in everyday parlance (e.g. "*. . . what we talked about was a kind of vision of what we might do . . .*").

In sum, there is a fair amount of fluidity surrounding the word "vision," and discussions of vision often conjure up different meanings for different people – even scholarly arguments often mix up different aspects of the notion and thus render the findings somewhat ambiguous. However, despite the somewhat equivocal nature of the term, we do not find any calls in the literature to abandon its use on account of it being too broad or vague. It will be argued in this book that there is good reason for this: the various layers and facets of the notion are ultimately interlinked as they are all connected to one of humanity's most remarkable capabilities, the "faculty of mental imagery." It is the desire to understand better this special faculty that has motivated the combined approach taken in the current book, namely to integrate considerations of science and theology, so let us begin the discussion by examining the potential benefits of this approach.

The complementary relationship between science and theology in understanding vision

My first encounter with the notion of vision occurred in my scientific research on the psychology of language learning,[6] and this encounter convinced me that vision was more than simply a metaphor to describe human imagination. I discovered that the concept of vision had concrete neuroscientific validity, as the brain uses virtually the same neural regions to generate mental images as it does to produce "real" images of what one actually sees.[7] Indeed, over the past three decades cognitive neuroscience has provided ample evidence that from the brain's perspective there is relatively little difference between *physically sensing* something (i.e. seeing, hearing, smelling, etc.) and *mentally simulating* the same sensation. Having completed a major

---

6 E.g. Dörnyei, "Future Self-Guides and Vision"; Dörnyei and Chan, "Motivation and Vision."
7 In their authoritative overview of cognitive neuroscience, Gazzaniga, Ivry and Mangun (*Cognitive Neuroscience*, 239) sum this up as follows: "The evidence provides a compelling case that mental imagery uses many of the same processes critical for perception. The sights in an image are likely to activate visual areas of the brain; the sounds, auditory areas; and the smells, olfactory areas."

research project examining the practical implications of vision in language education,[8] I came to the realisation that my findings could potentially also be relevant to theology and that, in fact, theology could provide further clarification of the concept of vision: while neuropsychology can speak about the distinctive and indeed remarkable human faculty of visualising imaginary pictures and scenes, theology can give meaning to this capability by linking it to God's created order. Scientific insights still remain useful for a theological understanding, though, as they can offer a coherent framework to accommodate various, rather fragmented theological considerations related to different aspects of visions, dreams and prophecy.

Thus, this book is based on the tenet that science and theology can offer different but complementary insights into the nature of God's creation, and the integrated approach adopted in the following chapters replicates my understanding of the fuller notion of vision by moving from the material realm (science) to the ethereal (theology). This is, in fact, not unlike how divine vision often operates: it draws on imagery that humans are familiar with in the physical world, but then shifts the receivers' attention from this material world to an alternative reality, thereby creating, in effect, an interface between the earthly and heavenly spheres.

The significance of vision

At the heart of almost every discussion of the significance of vision lies an observation summarised by Gregory Boyd as follows: "it's not so much what we intellectually believe is true that impacts us; it's what we experience as real,"[9] a principle that is reflected in everyday sayings such as "I'll believe it when I see it." As mentioned briefly earlier, the uniqueness of the faculty of vision is in its ability to create an experience of an envisaged reality that can be as vivid and life-like as the material reality that we perceive through our physical senses. This is explained by the fact that the brain uses virtually the same processing regions to generate the "imaginary" experience as for processing the concrete experience of the world. As a result, the alternative reality can have the same intensity of impact on humans as the physical reality of the material world.[10]

This unique imaginary faculty naturally lends itself to be utilised in *artistic expression*, and although this topic is beyond the scope of the current book, by way of illustration of this interrelationship of vision and art, here is what C. S. Lewis said about the creation of his famous *Narnia* series:[11]

---

8 Dörnyei and Kubanyiova, *Motivating Learners*.
9 Boyd, *Seeing Is Believing*, 12.
10 E.g. in a paper in the journal *Brain Research*, Decety and Grézes ("The Power of Simulation," 4) conclude, "One fascinating characteristic of human nature is our ability to consciously use our imagination to simulate reality as well as fictional worlds."
11 I am grateful to Sam Wong for drawing my attention to this quote.

All my seven Narnian books, and my three science fiction books, began with seeing pictures in my head. At first they were not a story, just pictures. The *Lion* [i.e. *The Lion, The Witch, and The Wardrobe*] all began with a picture of a Faun carrying an umbrella and parcels in a snowy wood. This picture had been in my mind since I was about sixteen. Then one day, when I was about forty, I said to myself: "Let's try to make a story about it." At first I had very little idea how the story would go. But then suddenly Aslan came bounding into it. . . . I don't know where the Lion came from or why He came. But once He was there He pulled the whole story together.[12]

The faculty of vision has also been utilised in *science* and *politics*. Chapters 1 and 2 will elaborate on scientific applications, but it might be interesting to note here as a preliminary illustration that while Albert Einstein was still a teenager, he repeatedly imagined himself chasing after a beam of light in space and visualised how the scene would look from this perspective. He recalled later that this thought experiment had played a decisive role in his development of the theory of special relativity.[13] Regarding politics, one of the most memorable examples of the application of vision was in a speech given by the Rev. Dr. Martin Luther King, Jr. about civil rights and racial equality in the 1960s. As will be further discussed later, at the end of this speech he departed from his prepared text and finished by describing an extended vision of a brighter future, punctuated with eight occurrences of the now legendary phrase, "*I have a dream.* . . ." His vision of an alternative future touched his hearers in a way that rational arguments, however convincing, could not have.

Finally, and most importantly for our current purpose, the existence of a dual sensory system in humans – consisting of outward physical senses on the one hand and an inner system of mentally simulated senses on the other – also has special *theological* relevance. The significance of the physical senses does not need any particular justification in view of the fact that humans were created to serve as stewards of material creation, and therefore it is clear that in order to be able to oversee the world around them, they need to receive ongoing multi-sensory (i.e. visual, auditory, tactile, gustatory and olfactory) stimuli. However, the internal senses are somewhat different in this respect in that they are not directly required for experiencing the physical environment. Yet, as will be argued in Chapters 3 and 4, the alternative sensory system is in fact equally important for the successful functioning of God's stewards, because the human ability to envisage and behold non-material reality opens up a further, mental, channel that enables humans to receive divine communication from the Creator. Indeed,

12 Lewis, *On Stories*, 53–54.
13 See, Norton, "Chasing the Light"; Robertson, *The Mind's Eye*, 89–90.

Chapter 3 will show that visions in the Bible almost always occur having this function, allowing prophets – and after Pentecost, also Christian believers in general – to receive direct messages from God; as William Arnold succinctly summarises, visions are "audiovisual means of communication between a heavenly being and an earthly recipient."[14]

Such an understanding of the faculty of vision is by no means new. As early as at the beginning of the 5th century, Augustine of Hippo submitted that "The one thing certain, which I think it is enough to insist on for the time being, is that there is a kind of *spiritual element* in us where the *likenesses of bodily things* [i.e. visions] are formed"[15] (emphasis added). In other words, and we shall see this later in more detail, Augustine believed that the faculty of internal vision is ultimately a "spiritual element" embedded in corporeal humans, and as such it resonates with the celestial realm. The thesis of my previous work on *Progressive Creation and the Struggles of Humanity in the Bible*[16] accentuated the declaration of Jesus Christ in John 6:17 that "My Father is still working, and I also am working," and the current book understands divine vision, as described in the Scriptures, as *one of the main vehicles of God's intervention in human history.* This belief is consistent with Karl Rahner's assertion that "the history of Christianity would be unthinkable without prophetic and visionary elements (in the broadest sense)."[17]

How is vision different from other related concepts?

Given the broad range of meanings that the term vision can subsume, it is important to distinguish the notion from other related concepts with which it has been linked – and often confused – in the past. We shall start by examining three terms – imagination, religious experience and revelation – that have frequently been used in biblical scholarship to include a visionary dimension. The section will then conclude with distinguishing "vision" from "mission" as used in the (church) leadership literature.

Vision and imagination

In a treatise on *imagination* within his work *On the Soul* (350 BC), Aristotle defined the notion in relation to "image" – as "the process by which we say that an image is presented to us"[18] – and, consequently, imagination and mental imagery have often been treated as equivalent terms in philosophy

---

14 Arnold, "Visions," 802.
15 Augustine, *On the Literal Meaning of Genesis*, 12.49 (p. 490).
16 Dörnyei, *Progressive Creation*.
17 Rahner, *Visions and Prophecies*, 15.
18 www.loebclassics.com/view/aristotle-soul/1957/pb_LCL288.159.xml. For a detailed discussion of Aristotle's conception of imagination, see Karnes, *Imagination*, 23–61; as she

and theology; as Nigel Thomas summarises, particularly prior to the 20th century, imagination was predominantly used "to name the faculty of image production (or the mental arena in which images appear),"[19] and this practice has remained prevalent also in some modern scholarship. For example, Garrett Green has defined imagination as a faculty that "makes present through images what is inaccessible to direct experience,"[20] and Colin McGinn declared, "I would suggest regarding the mind as centrally a device for imagining. We are *Homo imaginans*. It is the mental image and its various elaborations that sums up what the human most characteristically is."[21]

Representing a somewhat different perspective, Kevin Vanhoozer argues that "the imagination is not merely a factory for producing mental images,"[22] because the notion assumes particular importance "when we consider its verbal rather than pictorial application,"[23] especially when it is associated with creative language such as metaphors. As he further asserts, the Bible is replete with metaphors,[24] which is no accident given that perceiving the divine requires humans to relate the essentially unfathomable to the experiences and realities of their own world, which is precisely what metaphors achieve with great effectiveness. It is, then, the imagination which ultimately produces the creative link between the unfamiliar and the familiar, and therefore, Vanhoozer submits that "Disciples need imagination to stay awake to the reality of what is in Christ."[25] He also adds that "reading Scripture theologically further requires imagination, the faculty which makes sense of things, locating particular bits and pieces within larger patterns."[26] Indeed, if we understand imagination as the ability to go beyond reality, it is in itself an act of imagination to engage with the written text of Scripture and see the larger whole.

Vanhoozer's overall conclusion is that imagination is "a cognitive faculty for creating meaning through making and then verbalizing conceptual associations (i.e. likening)."[27] This understanding of a broad mental function has been supported by psychological research; in a recent review, for example, Luca Tateo has defined imagination as "a fundamental psychological higher function that elaborates meaning by linguistic and iconic signs,

---

concludes, Aristotle uses the notion for a wide range of purposes, "so wide that it is difficult to find a coherent theory of imagination at the heart of them" (p. 33).

19 Thomas, "Theories of Imagery," 207–208; see also Thomas, "The Multidimensional Spectrum of Imagination."
20 Green, *Imagining God*, 62.
21 McGinn, *Mindsight*, 5. Another example is Karnes's comprehensive book on *Imagination, Meditation, and Cognition in the Middle Ages*, where she states at the beginning, "The focus of this study is solely on mental images" (p. 17), which she then discusses as being subsumed under the notion of imagination.
22 Vanhoozer, "C. S. Lewis on the Imagination," 99.
23 Vanhoozer, "Imagination in Theology," 442.
24 Vanhoozer, *Pictures at a Theological Exhibition*, 28.
25 Vanhoozer, "C. S. Lewis on the Imagination," 104.
26 Vanhoozer, "Imagination in Theology," 442.
27 Vanhoozer, "C. S. Lewis on the Imagination," 99.

related to memory, fantasy and intelligence, playing a crucial role in scientific thinking, art, and societal change as well as in education and promotion of wellbeing."[28] In this sense, Tateo underlines, "it is distinct from fantasy, imagery and simulation, being the basic function underlying them".[29] In a similar vein, other scholars have used "imagination" as an umbrella-term that subsumes a long list of related phenomena such as creativity, originality, fantasy, innovation, inventiveness and idiosyncrasy, as well as a variety of mental activities such as supposing, pretending, thinking of possibilities, considering hypothetical options, conjuring up images, stories and projections of things not present, planning for and anticipating the future, and even thinking counterfactually.[30] In *The Oxford Handbook of the Development of Imagination*, Marjorie Taylor is thus right to conclude that various authors differ in their views of how to define imagination and its relation to mental imagery, creativity and memory.[31]

To summarise, there is no doubt that imagination is an important feature of the human mind, yet it is also clear that the faculty of vision is different from, although often contributing to, this higher mental function. The proposal that "imagination" in the broader sense is necessary for relating to God and the Scriptures is a convincing one; in fact, Paul Avis starts his book on *God and the Creative Imagination* by declaring, "My thesis in this book is that Christianity lives supremely from the imagination,"[32] and then proposes an understanding of imagination that is very close to the view of vision that was put forward earlier in the current work:

> My starting point is the conviction that divine revelation is given above all (though certainly not exclusively) in modes that are addressed to the human imagination, rather than to any other faculty (such as the analytical reason or the moral conscience).[33]

In the end, however, it was deemed best for the current book to avoid using imagination as a technical term for two main reasons. First, the attraction of the notion of "vision" is partly that it can be defined with consistency within a neuropsychological framework, whereas the semantic breadth of the term imagination defies such efforts, as illustrated for example by Trevor Hart:

> What is imagination? There is no single or simple answer to this question. . . . Having stopped and thought about those activities and

---

28 Tateo, "Just an Illusion?" 1
29 Ibid.
30 See e.g. Modell, *Imagination,* 110; Moulton and Kosslyn, "Imagining Predictions," 1279; Runco and Pina, "Imagination and Creativity," 379; Taylor, "Transcending Time," 9; Taylor et al., "Harnessing the Imagination," 429–430; Thomas, "Imagination."
31 Taylor, "Transcending Time," 9.
32 Avis, *God and the Creative Imagination,* 3.
33 Ibid.

phenomena that we intuitively associate with the imaginative, attempts to list its key contributions reveal its basic and pervasive influence on much if not most of what, humanly, we do in the world and experience of it.[34]

Second, in spite of the relevance of imagination to Christian thinking, the term itself is, strictly speaking, not biblical; as Alison Searle sums up, there is "no direct correlate in either Hebrew or Greek for our English word imagination. Various English translations of the Bible have rendered different words from the original by this term or its cognates, but they are not consistent."[35] In fact, Vanhoozer adds that not only is there no Hebrew or Greek biblical term for imagination, but the influential King James Version has actually created *prejudice* against the word by using it pejoratively[36] in contexts such as "imagination of the evil heart" (Jer 3:17), "wicked imaginations" (Prov 6:18) or "proud in the imagination of their hearts" (Luke 1:51).[37]

Vision and religious experience

When vision is used in the sense of seeing in the mind's eye (i.e. not as physical sight), the notion is often conflated with unique and out-of-the-ordinary human experiences that may accompany a vision; that is, when we hear that someone has "seen a vision," we normally assume this to be more than merely a mental picture. Rather, we suppose that the visionary experience was accompanied by some form of altered state of consciousness in the context of a "psychedelic" vision or a religious experience in spiritual contexts. There is no question that vision sometimes occurs as embedded within some unique physical experience; for example, in the Old Testament, Balaam is described as receiving a divine vision while in some kind of altered bodily state – "the oracle of one who hears the words of God, who sees the vision of the Almighty, who falls down, but with eyes uncovered" (Num 24:4 and 16) – and similarly, the prophet Daniel narrates that "So I was left alone to see this great vision. My strength left me, and my complexion grew deathly pale, and I retained no strength. Then I heard the sound of his words; and when I heard the sound of his words, I fell into a trance,[38] face to the ground" (Dan 10:8–9). In the New Testament, the Apostle Peter also "fell into a trance [*ékstasis*]" (Acts 10:10) when he received the momentous

---

34 Hart, "Imagination," 321.
35 Searle, *The Eyes of Your Heart*, 32–33. For a summary of the various Greek and Hebrew concepts related to imagination in the biblical corpus, as well as the different ways in which they have been translated into English, see ibid., 32–34.
36 Vanhoozer, *Pictures at a Theological Exhibition*, 19.
37 See also Gen 6:5; 8.21; Jer 3:7; 7:24; 9:14; 11:18; 13:10; 18:12; 23:17; Lam 3:60–61; Rom 1:21; 2 Cor 10:5.
38 The meaning of the Hebrew word (*râdam*) literally means "falling into heavy sleep," but the context shows that in this case it refers to more than ordinary sleep; this is further indicated by the fact that during the vision Daniel actually "stood up trembling" (Dan 10:12).

vision about eating unclean animals (Acts 10:9–16) which eventually led to the acceptance of Gentile believers into the emerging Christian Church.

Prophetic visions in the Bible are also often accompanied by some curious phraseology: on more than ten occasions in the Old Testament, we read that "the hand of the Lord" (e.g. Ezek 3:14) was on the prophets, and in many other instances the prophet was "in the Spirit" (e.g. Rev 1:10) or "the spirit of God came upon him" (e.g. Isa 61:1), which suggests to some scholars[39] that these phrases signify enhanced bodily states. David Aune makes an insightful point in this respect when he argues that although these expressions reveal little about the actual nature of the visionary state, they clearly mark "the onset of the revelatory state from the normal state of consciousness,"[40] thereby indirectly evidencing the existence of such a special state.

The close link between vision and religious experience has often hijacked the discussion of vision in the sense that typically it was the pros and cons related to "mystic experiences" that dominated the discourse. It is easy to see why this might happen, but it needs to be emphasised that from a scientific point of view, vision and altered states of consciousness are distinct phenomena. This issue will be further discussed in the next chapter, but it is important to address here briefly the source of the close association of the two notions. The link has an indirect neurological basis: since physical sight and imaginary vision are represented largely in the same neural region of the brain, the two sets of stimuli inevitably "compete" with each other in that they cannot occur at the same time, and physical sight can cancel out or weaken mental imagery. For this reason, sustained internal vision can more easily take place if one's physical perceptions are dimmed (e.g. in a dark and quiet place) or altogether suspended (e.g. in a dream state or in various forms of altered states of consciousness). In this sense, therefore, the various bodily states that are associated with the broad concept of "religious experience" may act as *facilitative conditions* for beholding vision, yet they are not prerequisites to it. Also, as Barbara Newman rightly points out, "Although the Bible from beginning to end is laced with visions, its writers showed little interest in the subjective experience of the visionary,"[41] and we may add that many genuine visionary states are *not* accompanied by any bodily symptoms at all.

Thus, it will be argued in Chapters 1 and 5 that there is no inextricable link between vision and altered bodily states, even though they sometimes occur together. This is important to stress, because in the past this co-occurrence has established a somewhat questionable reputation for the concept of vision in certain church circles (e.g. amongst Evangelicals) due to the subjective and unverifiable nature of religious experiences. If, however,

---

39 E.g. Pilch, *Flights of the Soul*, 33; Aune, "Trance," 886.
40 Aune, "Ecstasy," 15.
41 Newman, "Medieval Visionary Culture," 1.

we can move beyond this apprehension, the notion of vision can enrich several aspects of Christian life and church practice; for example, as will be elaborated upon in Chapter 6, vision has been utilised equally in Ignatian spirituality in the Catholic tradition and by prominent Evangelical church leaders such as John Piper, Andy Stanley and Rick Warren for the purpose of enhancing the effectiveness of leadership practices.

Vision and revelation

In 2 Corinthians 12:1, Paul speaks of visions and revelations as two closely related notions – "I will go on to visions [*optasia*] and revelations [*apokalypsis*] of the Lord" – and commentators have been divided as to whether the two words are used here as synonyms,[42] perhaps in the manner of a "hendiadys"[43] (i.e. "visionary revelations" or "revelatory visions"), or whether they mark some kind of a difference between the concepts, with revelation usually considered a wider category.[44] Elsewhere in Paul's writings, the two terms appear to be used interchangeably: in Galatians 1:12, for example, he states about the gospel that "I did not receive it from a human source, nor was I taught it, but I received it through a *revelation* of Jesus Christ" (emphasis added), and in Acts 26:19 he refers to what Jesus taught him as "the heavenly vision." The more general literature on the two concepts shows a similar ambiguity, with the words at times used interchangeably.[45] A helpful definition for divine revelation has been offered by Robert Yarbrough in the *New Dictionary of Biblical Theology*, referring to it as "the disclosure by God of truths at which people could not arrive without divine initiative and enabling,"[46] and such a disclosure would certainly include divine vision, as proposed by John Miller for example:

> In the Gospels, dreams/visions typically feature an irruption of the divine into human experience, offering some form of revelation to the recipient(s). They provide vivid imagery depicting God at work within the scenes of human history, and they evoke a broader sense of God at work behind the scenes of human history.[47]

42 E.g. Aune, "Vision," 994.
43 E.g. Lambrecht, *Second Corinthians*, 200.
44 E.g. Harris, "2 Corinthians," 531.
45 Packer ("Revelation," 1014) offers a good summary of the fluidity of the notion when he concludes, "when the Bible speaks of revelation, the thought intended is of God the Creator actively disclosing to men his power and glory, his nature and character, his will, ways and plans – in short, himself – in order that men may know him. The revelation vocabulary in both Testaments is a wide one, covering the ideas of making obscure things clear, bringing hidden things to light, showing signs, speaking words and causing the persons addressed to see, hear, perceive, understand and know."
46 Yarbrough, "Revelation," 732.
47 Miller, "Dreams and Visions," 218.

To avoid any unnecessary confusion, in the current work "revelation" will not be used as a technical term with a specific referent but rather as a spectrum of divine means of disclosure, leading to a range of outcomes, from intellectual illumination and guidance to eschatological insights.[48] In this sense, Aune is right in stating that vision is a "revelatory medium."[49] We shall return to this question in more detail in Chapter 3.

Vision and mission

Finally, there is a distinction to be made between vision as we have considered it previously in this introduction and the extended understanding of "vision" as referring to the picturing of a desired future, or in John Stott's words, "an imaginative perception of things, combining insight and foresight."[50] As we saw above, in the *British National Corpus* this sense of the word vision has the most occurrences, and in the Christian literature vision used as a sought-after future plan is often linked to the term "mission": for example, if we were to compare the vision statements and mission statements of various ministries, we would be hard put to be able to identify any real systematic difference. In the current book, however, the two terms will be used in a different way, with vision referring to an extended *image* and mission to an abstract *goal*. Malphurs and Penfold describe a mission as "a clear statement of where the organization is going," whereas the vision refers to "a snapshot of what it will look like when the church gets there."[51] The same distinction between vision and mission is also often made in psychology.[52] This distinction is not merely a terminological subtlety but concerns the core thesis of this book. Even when we talk about future aspirations, a vision has a strong *perceptual element*, that is, a picture-like quality;[53] Ira Levin's definition offers an excellent summary:

> Effective visions should describe a future world where the mission is advanced. . . . They should outline a rich and textual picture of what success looks like and feels like. Such visions paint a picture and tell a story. It is not enough to simply state where an organization is headed or what its general aspirations are. The vision should be so vivid as

48 See Dunn, "Biblical Concepts of Revelation," 14–15.
49 Aune, "Vision," 994.
50 Stott, *Issues Facing Christians*, 487.
51 Malphurs and Penfold, *Re:Vision*, 153.
52 E.g. Mirvis, Googins and Kinnicutt ("Vision, Mission, Values," 317) write in the journal *Organizational Dynamics*: "1. Vision is the 'What:' the picture of the future we seek to create. 2. Mission is the 'Why:' the organization's answer to why we exist (purpose)."
53 According to Berg ("Purpose and Goals in Visions," 3), "The definitions of company vision vary but they all contain elements of an ideal future state. Vision is a desired state of products, services and an organization that a leader wants to realize. It is an idyllic and distinctive representation of the future."

to enable the listener or reader to transport himself or herself to the future, so to speak, to witness it and experience it. This level of detailed description helps people understand how the future world is both similar to and different from the current one and what could be their potential role in it.[54]

The link between mental imagery and future vision will be further discussed in Chapter 2, with a special focus on the characteristics of effective vision statements.

How can vision enrich Christian life and ministry?

Over the past four decades, the notion of vision has become a central theme in the business world, because envisaging an attractive future has been found to be an effective tool for promoting human motivation and performance. Indeed, the success of legendary business leaders such as Steve Jobs or Walt Disney has typically been ascribed to their visionary capacity. The high value placed on vision in the marketplace has been verified by a solid body of research in business studies and organisational psychology, as well as by elaborate psychological models generated to explain the motivational impact of vision. No wonder, therefore, that the notion of vision has also been taken up in the literature on Christian leadership, especially in North American Protestant circles. Influential authors such as Aubrey Malphurs, John Maxwell, Andy Stanley and Rick Warren have argued that visionary leadership is a prerequisite to church growth and that, in fact, without it the church cannot prosper.

The current book is in agreement with the position that vision potentially has far-reaching relevance for Christian ministry, and intends to make a novel contribution in two ways. First, while the existing Christian literature has been effective in drawing on vision-related knowledge accumulated from business studies, it has not to the same extent interacted with the theoretical findings of psychology and cognitive science. It will be shown that a great deal of the neuropsychological knowledge of "mental imagery" – the term usually used to refer to vision – is transferrable to Christian contexts for the purpose of increasing the effectiveness of visionary thinking. Second, while the existing Christian literature typically discusses vision at the level of church organisation and leadership (although see Chapter 6 for exceptions), the current book will place greater emphasis on how *individual* believers can utilise vision to given direction to their own Christian walk. In this way, the discussion will share much in common with, and will draw extensively on, scholarship in the Catholic church regarding the notion of "Election" within Ignatian spirituality (see Chapter 6).

54 Levin, "Vision Revisited," 95.

The structure and possible uses of this book

In order to prepare the ground for the discussion of the practical implications of vision for the Christian life – which is the primary purpose of this work – the book will first offer a survey of the various scientific findings relevant to vision (Chapters 1 and 2), followed by two chapters (Chapters 3 and 4) examining biblical vision through the analysis of visionary experiences reported in the Scriptures. Chapter 5 looks at the critical question of how the divine origin of a visionary message can be ascertained, particularly in view of the vulnerabilities that beset the divine-human communication channel. Chapter 6 surveys the two most established uses of vision in Christian traditions: cultivated vision (including Ignatian spirituality) and visionary leadership practices. Then, the final two chapters (Chapters 7 and 8) provide practical guidelines on how vision can help believers to discern God's plans for them and how they can appropriately strengthen and sustain the divine purpose they have perceived in their everyday lives.

The eight chapters are relatively self-contained and each concludes with a comparatively jargon-free summary. As such, the time-pressed reader is able to take a "pick-and-mix" approach to reading the material, possibly even beginning with the final two practical chapters or the Conclusion. In other words, it is possible to use this book as a reference work to dip in and out of, with the frequent cross-references pointing to other parts of the material that might also be of interest. Such a selective approach may also be recommended in the light of the wide range of material covered: readers coming to the text with different backgrounds may well find some sections too technical or too detailed, in which case they can receive a quick overview from the chapter summary and then move on to the parts that are more relevant to them.

References

Arnold, William T. 1996. "Visions." In *Evangelical Dictionary of Biblical Theology*, edited by Walter A. Elwell, 802–03. Grand Rapids, MI: Baker Books.

Augustine of Hippo. 2002. *On the Literal Meaning of Genesis* (in: *On Genesis*). Translated by Edmund Hill. New York: New City Press, 415.

Aune, David E. 1988. "Ecstasy." In *The International Standard Bible Encyclopedia, Revised*, edited by Geoffrey W. Bromiley, 14–16. Grand Rapids, MI: Eerdmans.

Aune, David E. 1988. "Trance." In *The International Standard Bible Encyclopedia, Revised*, edited by Geoffrey W. Bromiley, 886. Grand Rapids, MI: Eerdmans.

Aune, David E. 1988. "Vision." In *The International Standard Bible Encyclopedia, Revised*, edited by Geoffrey W. Bromiley, 993–94. Grand Rapids, MI: Eerdmans.

Avis, Paul. 1999. *God and the Creative Imagination: Metaphor, Symbol and Myth in Religion and Theology*. London: Routledge.

Berg, Jodi L. 2015. "The Role of Personal Purpose and Personal Goals in Symbiotic Visions." *Frontiers in Psychology* 6, no. 443: 1–13.

Boyd, Gregory A. 2004. *Seeing Is Believing: Experience Jesus through Imaginative Prayer*. Grand Rapids, MI: Baker Books.

Decety, Jean, and Julie Grèzes. 2006. "The Power of Simulation: Imagining One's Own and Other's Behavior." *Brain Research* 1079: 1–14.

Dörnyei, Zoltán. 2014. "Future Self-Guides and Vision." In *The Impact of Self-Concept on Language Learning*, edited by K. Csizér and M. Magid, 7–18. Bristol: Multilingual Matters.

Dörnyei, Zoltán. 2018. *Progressive Creation and Humanity's Struggles in the Bible: A Canonical Narrative Interpretation*. Eugene, OR: Pickwick.

Dörnyei, Zoltán, and Letty Chan. 2013. "Motivation and Vision: An Analysis of Future L2 Self Images, Sensory Styles, and Imagery Capacity across Two Target Languages." *Language Learning* 63, no. 3: 437–62.

Dörnyei, Zoltán, and Maggie Kubanyiova. 2014. *Motivating Learners, Motivating Teachers: Building Vision in the Language Classroom*. Cambridge: Cambridge University Press.

Dunn, James D. G. 1997. "Biblical Concepts of Revelation." In *Divine Revelation*, edited by Paul Avis, 1–22. Eugene, OR: Wipf and Stock.

Gazzaniga, Michael S., Richard B. Ivry, and George R. Mangun. 2002. *Cognitive Neuroscience: The Biology of the Mind*. New York: W. W. Norton.

Green, Garrett. 1989. *Imagining God: Theology and the Religious Imagination*. New York: Harper and Row.

Harris, Murray J. 2008. "2 Corinthians." In *The Expositor's Bible Commentary: Romans – Galatians (Revised Edition)*, edited by Tremper III Longman and David E. Garland, 239–414. Grand Rapids, MI: Zondervan.

Hart, Trevor A. 2005. "Imagination." In *Dictionary for Theological Interpretation of the Bible*, edited by Kevin J. Vanhoozer, 321–23. Grand Rapids, MI: Baker Academic.

Karnes, Michelle. 2011. *Imagination, Meditation, and Cognition in the Middle Ages*. Chicago: University of Chicago Press.

Lambrecht, Jan. *Second Corinthians*. Sacra Pagina 8. Collegeville, MN.: Liturgical Press, 1999.

Levin, Ira M. 2000. "Vision Revisited: Telling the Story of the Future." *Journal of Applied Behavioral Science* 36, no. 1: 91–107.

Lewis, C. S. 2002. *On Stories and Other Essays in Literature*. Orlando, FL: Harcourt.

Malphurs, Aubrey, and Gordon E. Penfold. 2014. *Re:Vision: The Key to Transforming Your Church*. Grand Rapids, MI: Baker Books.

McGinn, Colin. 2004. *Mindsight: Image, Dream, Meaning*. Cambridge, MA: Harvard University Press.

Miller, John B. F. 2013. "Dreams and Visions." In *Dictionary of Jesus and the Gospels; Second Edition* edited by Joel B. Green, Jeannine K. Brown and Norman Perrin, 216–18. Downers Grove, IL: IVP Academic.

Mirvis, Philip, Bradley Googins, and Sylvia Kinnicutt. 2010. "Vision, Mission, Values: Guideposts to Sustainability." *Organizational Dynamics* 39: 316–24.

Modell, Arnold H. 2003. *Imagination and the Meaningful Brain*. Cambridge, MA: MIT Press.

Moulton, Samuel T., and Stephen M. Kosslyn. 2009. "Imagining Predictions: Mental Imagery as Mental Emulation." *Philosophical Transactions of the Royal Society B* 364: 1273–80.

Newman, Barbara. 2005. "What Did It Mean to Say "I Saw"? The Clash between Theory and Practice in Medieval Visionary Culture." *Speculum* 80, no. 1: 1–43.

Norton, John D. 2013. "Chasing the Light: Einstein's Most Famous Thought Experiment." In *Thought Experiments in Science, Philosophy, and the Arts*, edited by

Mélanie Frappier, Letitia Meynell and James Robert Brown, 123–40. London: Routledge.

Packer, J. I. 1996. "Revelation." In *New Bible Dictionary*, edited by I. Howard Marshall, A. R. Millard, J. I. Packer and D. J. Wiseman, 1014–16. Downers Grove, IL: InterVarsity Press.

Pilch, John J. 2011. *Flights of the Soul: Visions, Heavenly Journeys, and Peak Experiences in the Biblical World*. Grand Rapids, MI: Eerdmans.

Rahner, Karl. 1963. *Visions and Prophecies*. Translated by Charles H. Henkey and Richard Strachan. Freiburg: Herder.

Robertson, Ian. 2002. *The Mind's Eye: An Essential Guide to Boosting Your Mental Power*. London: Bantam Books.

Runco, Mark A., and Jeremy Pina. 2013. "Imagination and Personal Creativity." In *The Oxford Handbook of the Development of Imagination*, edited by Marjorie Taylor, 379–86. Oxford: Oxford University Press.

Searle, Alison. 2008. *'The Eyes of Your Heart': Literary and Theological Trajectories of Imagining Biblically*. Milton Keynes: Paternoster.

Stott, John. 2011. *Issues Facing Christians Today*. 4th ed. Grand Rapids, MI: Zondervan.

Tateo, Luca. 2015. "Just an Illusion? Imagination as Higher Mental Function." *Psychology and Psychotherapy* 5, no. 6: 1–6.

Taylor, Marjorie. 2013. "Transcending Time, Place, and/or Circumstance: An Introduction." In *The Oxford Handbook of the Development of Imagination*, edited by Marjorie Taylor, 3–10. Oxford: Oxford University Press.

Taylor, Shelley E., Lien B. Pham, Inna D. Rivkin, and David A. Armor. 1998. "Harnessing the Imagination: Mental Simulation, Self-Regulation, and Coping." *American Psychologist* 53, no. 4: 429–39.

Thomas, Nigel J. T. 1999. "Are Theories of Imagery Theories of Imagination? An Active Perception Approach to Conscious Mental Content." *Cognitive Science* 23, no. 2: 207–45.

Thomas, Nigel J. T. 2004. "Imagination." In *Dictionary of philosophy of mind*, edited by Eric Hochstein. https://sites.google.com/site/minddict/imagination.

Thomas, Nigel J. T. 2014. "The Multidimensional Spectrum of Imagination: Images, Dreams, Hallucinations, and Active, Imaginative Perception." *Humanities* 3: 132–84.

van der Helm, R. 2009. "The Vision Phenomenon: Towards a Theoretical Underpinning of Visions of the Future and the Process of Envisioning." *Futures* 41: 96–104.

Vanhoozer, Kevin J. 2014. "In Bright Shadow: C. S. Lewis on the Imagination for Theology and Discipleship." In *The Romantic Rationalist: God, Life, and Imagination in the Work of C. S. Lewis*, edited by John Piper and David Mathis, 81–104. Wheaton, IL: Crossway.

Vanhoozer, Kevin J. 2016a. "Imagination in Theology." In *New Dictionary of Theology: Historic and Systematic*, edited by Martin Davie, Tim Grass, Stephen R. Holmes, John McDowell and T. A. Noble, 441–43. Downers Grove, IL: IVP Academic.

Vanhoozer, Kevin J. 2016b. *Pictures at a Theological Exhibition: Scenes of the Church's Worship, Witness and Wisdom*. Downers Grove, IL: IVP Academic.

Yarbrough, R. W. 2000. "Revelation." In *New Dictionary of Biblical Theology*, edited by T. Desmond Alexander and Brian S. Rosner, 732–38. Leicester: InterVarsity Press.

1 Vision and mental imagery in science

It was stated in the Introduction that vision is a remarkable built-in human faculty that can assign reality status to things that humans conceive only through their internal rather than their physical senses. It was also argued that this capacity is due in part to the brain being hard-wired to process physical perception (of the world) and mental imagery (e.g. internal vision) in the same neural regions, using similar processing mechanisms.[1] This chapter will elaborate on these claims by offering a brief overview of the relevant neuroscientific research with regard to five broad themes:

- The definition and significance of mental imagery.
- The neurobiological mechanism underlying mental imagery and its role in human cognitive functioning.
- The different sources, types and modalities of mental imagery.
- The interaction between the external and the internal senses, and the optimal conditions for mental imagery.
- The relationship between mental imagery and altered states of consciousness.

The discussion of these points will serve to provide a foundation for the next chapter to build on as it reviews the main applications of vision in psychology, sports and business management, ultimately drawing lessons that are transferrable to Christian contexts.

What is mental imagery and why is it important?

Cattaneo and Silvanto define "mental imagery" – the term typically used in cognitive science to refer to vision – "as a quasi-perceptual experience occurring in the absence of perceptual input."[2] *Quasi-perceptual experience* in this definition means that the imagery involves a mental representation

---

1 Although mental imagery is not a fully uniform entity (see e.g. Kosslyn and Rabin, "Imagery," 388), the various forms of internal vision share sufficient common ground to allow us to talk about "mental imagery" in general.
2 Cattaneo and Silvanto, "Mental Imagery," 220.

in the brain that is similar to the representation of actually seeing with the eye, however, *without* any external sensory input. As mentioned earlier, this faculty is well known to human experience, and most people would readily understand the concept of "seeing in the mind's eye," as described in Shakespeare's Hamlet.[3] The widespread familiarity with the notion of vision is partly due to the fact that mental imagery is closely associated with another common human behaviour, *daydreaming*. Eric Klinger's seminal psychological research in this area reveals that various forms of daydreaming are a common part of our mental activity, with as much as half of human thought potentially qualifying for it.[4] Our daydreams are often visual, and, interestingly, although they appear spontaneously – for example, when we are doing a monotonous task – we do have a certain amount of control over them in that we can influence not only when to stop and start daydreaming but we can also to some extent determine the content. The same thing, of course, cannot be said about the equally common experience of mental imagery: *night-time dreaming*.

The importance of mental imagery begins in childhood, when the role of fantasy and imagination is prominent in children's cognitive development. Indeed, it might be argued that they are an indispensable part of play, where children often create intricate worlds of make-believe.[5] This does in fact continue throughout education; as early as the end of the 19th century, the eminent American philosopher and educational reformer, John Dewey (1859–1952), declared that the central issue in education is *image-formation*:

> I believe that the image is the great instrument of instruction. What a child gets out of any subject presented to him is simply the images which he himself forms with regard to it. . . . I believe that much of the time and attention now given to the preparation and presentation of lessons might be more wisely and profitably expended in training the child's power of imagery and in seeing to it that he was continually forming definite, vivid, and growing images of the various subjects with which he comes in contact in his experience.[6]

Dewey's views have since received ample endorsement in psychology. For example, as we shall see later in detail, Allan Paivio's "dual coding theory" stipulates that human cognition involves the activity of two distinct subsystems, a verbal system specialised for dealing directly with language and a nonverbal (imagery) system specialised for dealing with non-linguistic objects and events.[7] Accordingly, information can be processed either verbally

3 Shakespeare, *Hamlet*, Act 1, Scene 2.
4 For an overview, see Klinger, "Daydreaming and Fantasizing."
5 See e.g. Segal, "Possible Selves," 83.
6 Dewey, "My Pedagogic Creed," 79–80.
7 Paivio, *Mental Representations*.

or visually, and to offer a quick illustration of this duality, if we ask people to think of, say, a carrot, most of us would not be able to help seeing at least a glimpse of orange colour. This indicates that information is stored in our memory also in a pictorial format, which explains in turn the beneficial impact of imagery on memory functions as well as other aspects of human cognitive performance – after all, as the saying goes, a picture is worth a thousand words!

The importance of vision does not in any way recede in adulthood; it can affect every aspect of our lives. Indeed, some of the greatest contributions and discoveries in the arts and sciences have been made through the use of mental imagery. As was already mentioned in the Introduction, C. S. Lewis, for example, created his famous Narnia series starting out from images in his head, and Albert Einstein developed his theory of relativity from a vision he had when he was 16. In a letter written to French mathematician Jacques Hadamard, Einstein explicitly stated:

> The words or the language, as they are written or spoken, do not seem to play any role in my mechanism of thought. The psychical entities which seem to serve as elements in thought are certain signs and more or less clear images which can be "voluntarily" reproduced and combined.[8]

Another powerful illustration of what can be achieved through the internal senses, this time through the auditory modality, concerns the composer Ludwig van Beethoven (1770–1827), who began to lose his hearing at the age of 26 and yet composed some of his best-known works (including his Ninth Symphony) when he was totally deaf, thereby providing evidence that hearing in the head – that is, "in the mind's ear" – can reach unprecedented subtlety.

While examples of how prominent artists and scientists utilised mental imagery for their creative work underscore the potential significance of vision, perhaps vision's most remarkable role in human life is one that most ordinary people can experience, namely *envisioning the future*. Research indicates that people spend a great deal of time conjuring up images of possible future scenarios and selves – both desired ones and feared ones – and there is robust evidence that this work of the imagination has powerful consequences; in Hazel Markus's words, it can help "to energize actions and to buffer the current self from everyday dragons and many less overt indignities as well."[9] Images of hoped-for future states have considerable motivational power, and Chapter 2 will describe the psychological theory of "possible selves" that explains how this mental energy source can be harnessed. As a result, Jerome Singer is right in declaring in his seminal book

8 Hadamard, *The Psychology of Invention*, 142.
9 Markus, "Foreword," xii.

on the subject that "Our capacity for imagery and fantasy can indeed give us a kind of control over possible futures!"[10]

The significance of mental imagery is also revealed when we consider its possible harmful impact. Mental images often play a distressing role in mental disorders such as phobias, post-traumatic stress disorder or schizophrenia, potentially causing paralysing fear, intrusive flashbacks of past failures and trauma, and even suicidal thoughts. In fact, some scholars believe that phobias are in effect disorders of imagery control,[11] and Singer argues that "the ruminations and repetitive thoughts of depressives, the chronically anxious, and the obsessed are reflections, in part, of a failure to develop the rich and varied imagery skills . . . [of] positive constructive daydreaming."[12] These skills, as mentioned before, usually develop in childhood, but Singer maintains that they can also be trained in adults through psychotherapy. These considerations suggest that human wellbeing can at least in part be attributed to healthy visionary functioning, a claim that chimes with a passage in the Beatitudes where Jesus declares of the (spiritual) eye, "The eye is the lamp of the body. So, if your eye is healthy, your whole body will be full of light; but if your eye is unhealthy, your whole body will be full of darkness" (Matt 6:22–23).

Singer is not alone in proposing that the power of imagery can be turned to therapeutic use. It is a well-demonstrated fact that mental visualisation can influence bodily functioning, including such basic functions as heart rate and blood flow, thereby suggesting that it could become an avenue for potent healing.[13] While it is true that many of the imagery-healing methods described on the Internet or in the popular media lack sufficient research foundation, as Ian Robertson rightly concludes, "your state of mind has profound effects on how well your body can fight off the viruses, bacteria, and dangerous cells that moment to moment are gnawing at the cage of our immunity."[14] The use of mental imagery can indeed create the right frame of mind to help combat several health issues (e.g. migraine, asthma, bronchitis and allergies) and manage mental conditions (e.g. fear, anxiety, stress and depression).

As a final illustration of the potency of mental imagery, let us turn to what some would perhaps consider a surprising example in this context: professional sports. As will be shown in the next chapter, sport psychology has been particularly active over the past two decades utilising visualisation techniques to enhance athletes' performance. One classic study of mental practice in golfing describes well the relevance of vision in this area: in 1985, Woolfolk, Parrish and Murphy carried out a fascinating investigation into the effect of imagery instruction on putting a golf ball, which is a simple

10 Singer, *Imagery in Psychotherapy*, 128.
11 See Baars, *Theater of Consciousness*, 76; Ji et al., "Emotional Mental Imagery," 704.
12 Singer, *Imagery in Psychotherapy*, 168.
13 See e.g. Katz. "Mental Imagery," 190.
14 Robertson, *The Mind's Eye*, 177.

motor skill accuracy task.[15] They asked some college students to imagine the backswing and putting stroke, with half of them visualising the ball going into the cup (i.e. positive imagery), while the other half imagined the ball narrowly missing the cup (i.e. negative imagery). There was also a control group who putted without instructions. The golfers then participated in a ten-putt trial on each of six consecutive days. The results were dramatic: over the six days the scores of the participants in the control group (i.e. no imagery) showed a level of improvement of around 10% that one would expect as a result of practice; in contrast, the golfers who exercised positive imagery improved by around 30%, while members of the negative imagery group actually got worse over the six-day period by as much as 20%! It would be difficult to find a more convincing illustration of the potential impact of mental visualisation on human activity.

The neurobiological foundation of vision

Mental imagery, as defined earlier, is the perception of an image when the source of the stimulus is not present. As Moulton and Kosslyn explain, such mental representations quite remarkably preserve the perceptible proper-ties of the stimulus by producing a realistic image.[16] The similarity between physical sensation and the forming of mental images was noticed by the famous 19th century American psychologist, William James (1842–1910), who also speculated as to whether the two processes could share the same regions of the brain.[17] The key question in this respect is posed by Gazzaniga and his colleagues as follows: "When we imagine our beachside sunset, are we activating the same neural pathways and performing the same internal operations as when we gaze upon such a scene with our eyes?"[18] It took almost a century to develop the necessary technology – most importantly, neuroimaging – to be able to assess this matter scientifically, but research over the past decade has increasingly confirmed that optical vision and vis-ual imagery utilise similar neural circuitry, activating about two thirds of the same brain areas.[19]

The overlap between visual perception and internal vision has been stud-ied extensively in neuropsychology and cognitive neuroscience, using a vari-ety of cutting-edge research tools and designs. For instance, in one study utilising functional MRI (i.e. a brain scan monitoring the change in blood flow), Meister and colleagues compared music performance and music imagery.[20] They found a strong overlap in the parts of the brain that were

15 Woolfolk, Parrish and Murphy, "Positive and Negative Imagery."
16 Moulton and Kosslyn, "Imagining Predictions," 1273.
17 See Modell, *Imagination,* 109.
18 Gazzaniga et al., *Cognitive Neuroscience,* 237.
19 Kosslyn et al., "Bridging Psychology and Biology," 342.
20 Meister et al., "Playing Piano in the Mind."

activated when the participants played music on a silent keyboard and when they imagined playing the same music without any actual finger movement. This was but one confirmation of the interrelated nature of motor execution and motor imagery, and other research has also found that the production of an action and imagining the same action share a number of common mental operations and rely upon common neural structures.[21]

According to Cattaneo and Silvanto's authoritative review of the psychology of mental imagery, arguably the strongest single piece of evidence indicating an overlap between the neural basis of visual perception and imagery was offered by Kreiman, Koch and Fried in the journal *Nature*.[22] These scholars examined single imagery neurons, which is a rare and difficult enterprise because it requires an "invasive" procedure of planting electrodes in the brain; for this reason, single neuron studies can only be done during surgery (e.g. when treating brain tumours or epilepsy).[23] Kreiman and his colleagues found a significant number of neurons in four brain regions that were activated *both* by visual and imaginary stimuli, which suggests "a common substrate for the processing of incoming visual information and visual recall."[24] In other words, mental imagery was found to be sensory in nature.

Despite the unquestionable commonalities between imagery and perception, we must stress that the two mental representations are not indistinguishable. It was already mentioned that the overlap between the perceptual and the imaginative domains is not total, and studies of patients with brain damage have also shown cases where the lesion resulted in a loss of mental imagery without a corresponding loss of perception and vice versa.[25] In most situations the brain *can* distinguish between physical perception and mental imagery, and in fact when this fails to happen, for example in some types of schizophrenia, it is regarded as a symptom of a mental dysfunction.[26] Thus, in normal cases, an imagined action does not activate our muscles like a real behavioural impulse does, although sometimes a particularly strong imagined impulse might lead to involuntary muscle movement. On balance, Robertson is right that "it is a miracle that we can – mostly – tell apart the mental image's firing of brain cells from the activity of near-identical sets of brain cells registering the outside world."[27] Of course, as he also reminds us, this does not happen in certain states, for example in dreaming or under hypnosis (an issue that we shall further examine later).

Thus, it is safe to conclude that human beings are hard-wired to generate, receive, behold and manipulate vision, and research shows that this faculty

21 See e.g. Decety and Grézes, "The Power of Simulation," 7.
22 Kreiman, Koch and Fried, "Imagery Neurons."
23 Fried et al., "Single Neuron Studies," 2.
24 Kreiman et al., "Imagery Neurons," 358.
25 Brogaard and Gatzia, "The Mental Imagery Debate," 1.
26 Robertson, *The Mind's Eye*, 73.
27 Ibid., 229.

is not a special skillset restricted to a selected few, but a generic feature of the whole human species. Moreover, this faculty is not learned but rather something we are born with, as evidenced by the fact that even people who are congenitally blind, that is, who have never experienced sight, are able to visualise to some extent. Helder Bértolo reports convincing evidence that blind people can create powerful mental images that have a lot in common with visual images;[28] for example, several blind subjects reported that when they sign their names they do not use a memorised set of movements but rather "visualise" their signature and reproduce it. Interestingly, one of Bértolo's participants revealed that during dreams he had experienced visual images, but he added that he was generally reluctant to share these experiences with others because his revelation typically met with disbelief.[29]

Vision and human mental functioning

It is true to say that not only are human beings hard-wired to be able to generate and behold vision, but this very faculty of visualisation also forms an integral part of higher order mental functioning in general. Aristotle claimed that "The soul never thinks without a mental image [*phantasma*],"[30] and contemporary psychology has confirmed that imagery plays an essential role in several aspects of thinking. There are two influential theories in cognitive psychology that illustrate this point well: Allan Paivio's *dual coding theory* (briefly mentioned earlier) and Alan Baddeley's concept of the *working memory*.

- *Dual coding theory*. Paivio was initially interested in the "mnemonic" benefits of imagery – that is, the use of imagery as a memory aid (a method employed to great effect by magicians) – but his research expanded into a more comprehensive theory of memory and cognition. His main finding was the realisation that cognition is made up of two interacting mental subsystems, *verbal* and *nonverbal/perceptual*, with mental imagery playing a central role in the second. In concrete terms, this means that people process information and store it in their memory in two different formats, one of which utilises pictorial codes.[31] This

---

28 Bértolo, "Visual Imagery Without Visual Perception," 183–184; see also Robertson, *The Mind's Eye*, 73–74. As will be discussed in more detail later, mental imagery also involves modalities other than visual (e.g. auditory), and research has established that congenitally blind people use the visual cortex of their brain to process different kinds of information such as auditory, tactile and haptic images. In this way, Bértolo concludes, they can process other sensory modalities "to integrate these inputs via the visual system to produce concepts capable of graphical representation" (p. 183).

29 Bértolo, "Visual Imagery Without Visual Perception," 184.

30 Aristotle, *De Anima*, III, 7; www.loebclassics.com/view/aristotle-soul/1957/pb_LCL288.177.xml?readMode=recto

31 As Paivio (*Mental Representations*, 53–54) explains, the pictorial system's critical functions include "the analysis of scenes and the generation of mental images (both functions

is evidenced by the fact that we can recall with ease pictures, sounds, smells and even tastes from our memory, and equally, certain pictures, sounds and smells that we encounter may trigger up memories of the past. The existence of the two parallel processing systems suggests that the combined and coordinated use of the two would result in enhanced cognitive performance, and this has indeed been found to be the case.[32]

- *Working memory* is a popular concept in psychology, referring to the "temporary storage and manipulation of information that is assumed to be necessary for a wide range of complex cognitive activities."[33] In Baddeley's model, originally proposed in the 1970s, the construct of working memory includes three main components: an attentional control system called the "central executive," as well as two subsystems, the "visuospatial sketchpad" and the "phonological loop," representing a visual and a verbal component.[34]

The parallels between Paivio's and Baddeley's theories on long-term memory (Paivio) and working memory (Baddeley) are clear in that both contain a prominent dimension whereby visual information is represented and manipulated. Recent research has begun to integrate not only these two conceptual systems but also the neuropsychological study of mental imagery.[35]

Sources, modalities and types of vision

Given the widespread presence of imagery in various human mental activities, we should expect to find a variety of different sources and types of vision, and this is indeed the case. This variety of visionary experiences will have direct implications for the theological understanding of divine vision.

Sources of mental imagery

A unique quality of mental imagery is that it forms an interface between the conscious and nonconscious parts of the self.[36] In other words, vision opens

---

encompassing other sensory modalities in addition to visual)." Reviewing the significance of this proposal, Pearson and Kosslyn ("Ending the Imagery Debate," 10089) underline the theory's importance in recognising that humans do not rely only on "language-like 'propositional' representations" (i.e. meaning that can be expressed in verbal statements), but also on information "stored in a depictive, pictorial format."

32 Pearson and Kosslyn, "Ending the Imagery Debate," 10089.
33 Baddeley, "Working Memory and Language," 189.
34 The visuospatial sketchpad is responsible for integrating spatial, visual and kinesthetic information into a unified representation, and the phonological loop is concerned with the temporary storage of verbal and acoustic information. See e.g. Baddeley and Andrade, "Working Memory and the Vividness of Imagery," 127.
35 Pearson et al., "Mental Imagery," 593–94; see also Cattaneo et al., "Working Memory and Imagery," 111–113; Richardson, *Imagery,* 138.
36 Thomas, *Mental Imaging in Counselling and Psychotherapy,* 3.

up a channel through which images from the subconscious can reach our conscious attention (which is best evidenced during dreaming). While such pictures sometimes pop into our minds spontaneously, at other times we can consciously conjure them up by directing our minds to create a fantasy, and we can also "discipline" our mind to get back on task when we are aware of drifting into daydreaming. Psychologists have been wondering about the origins of these images that emerge in the mind, and the standard scholarly answer has been that the various pictures arise either as direct imports of visual memories or as modified versions of these. In other words, psychologists maintain that the source of vision can be found in one's memory and that a mental image therefore involves *re-experiencing* a version of a stored stimulus or some novel combination of several stimuli.[37]

However, as early as the 1970s in one of the seminal works popularising vision, authors Mike and Nancy Samuels highlighted another form of vision – which they called "hallucination" – in which the person seeing the image believes its source to be external to him/herself.[38] That is, although cognitive neuroscience has not engaged with this matter, in popular culture there has been a belief that some images are sourced by external agents (e.g. spiritual forces). As we shall see in the last section of this chapter, historical anthropology has established that the vast majority of known cultures in the past have subscribed to this view and have experimented with "altered states of consciousness" to induce visionary states intentionally.

Modalities of vision

Even if we put aside the question of possible external origins of some images, visionary experiences display considerable diversity. The most obvious differences lie in the *modality* of vision, which refers to the different senses that are simulated mentally. Just as we can "see in the mind's eye," we can also "hear in the head" (a phenomenon that is sometimes called "audition"), and if we imagine biting into a piece of lemon, our teeth clench and we grimace because of the simulated sour taste in our mind. Thus, mental imagery can occur in any sensory modality, not purely the visual, even though when people report visionary experiences, they will usually start doing it using visual terms.[39] Having said that, auditions are also common,[40] because people frequently recall or imagine conversations they have had or are planning to have with someone. Interestingly, Robertson reports that when people rate the vividness of their imagery in the various senses, the sense of smell comes first, followed by taste.[41] In sport psychology, 'motor imagery' (or kinesthetic imagery) has particular relevance, because it concerns the

37 Pearson et al., "Mental Imagery," 590.
38 Samuels and Samuels, *Seeing with the Mind's Eye*, 50.
39 Hall et al., *Guided Imagery*, 7.
40 Pearson et al., "Assessing Mental Imagery," 6.
41 Robertson, *The Mind's Eye*, 66.

bodily sensations of action, allowing athletes to rehearse certain movement sequences mentally.[42]

It may be concluded regarding all these different types of imagery – along with modalities not yet discussed at length, such as tactile (touch), olfactory (smell) and gustatory (taste) – that neuroscientific research has replicated the same observations about them as about visual images, namely that there is a partial overlap of the neural networks processing them and their physical counterparts. For example a smell and an imagined smell are represented in similar regions in the brain.[43]

Types of mental imagery

The fact that human beings have the ability to simulate mentally any of their senses allows them to generate a rich source of mental scenarios: these can involve not only recalling what has happened in the past, but also envisaging hypothetical scenarios and fantasy scenes, as well as a mixture of real and hypothetical events such as replaying an argument and imagining what one should have said.[44] The following are some common forms of mental imagery: retrieving and reliving memories; visualising written narratives (e.g. novels); counterfactual thinking (i.e. imagining a counterfactual scenario such as Hungary winning the football world cup); imagining possible futures (which will be a central theme of the next chapter); daydreaming and fantasising.

One item on the list may be conspicuous by its absence: dreaming. This is not because dreaming does not include mental imagery; on the contrary: neuroimaging research by Tomoyasu Horikawa and his Japanese colleagues reported recently in *Science Magazine* has confirmed that the vivid visual content experienced by the sleeping dreamer is represented by the same neural substrate as observed during waking perception of mental imagery.[45] The reason why dreams did not fit neatly into the list is that the imagery in their case occurs while the dreamers are in a state in which they do not exercise consciousness. We do not consciously generate our dreams, even though they may be closely related to one's waking fantasies as well as recent thoughts and experiences (e.g. TV programmes, books, Internet sites).[46] Imagery-rich unconscious states can also be achieved by other means, for example by the use of psychedelic drugs such as LSD, which takes us to the broader subject of how mental imagery is related to what are usually called "altered states of consciousness" (ASC). In the concluding section of this chapter, we shall examine this topic in more detail, but in order to be able to fully

42 See e.g. Cumming and Ste-Marie, "Imagery Training," 284; Robertson, *The Mind's Eye*, 67.
43 Cattaneo and Silvanto, "Mental Imagery," 225.
44 Taylor et al., "Harnessing the Imagination," 430.
45 Horikawa et al., "Visual Imagery During Sleep," 639.
46 Singer, *Imagery in Psychotherapy*, 177.

appreciate the nature of the link between vision and exceptional experiential states such as dreams or trances, we first need to address another important issue, the *competition* between the external and the internal senses and the implications of this competition for the *optimal conditions* for experiencing mental imagery.

The competition between the physical and mental senses, and the optimal conditions for experiencing mental imagery

The reason that there is a competition between the external and the internal senses is straightforward: because physical perceptions and mental imagery are processed largely in the same neural substrate of the brain, people cannot experience both fully at the same time. In this respect, the two types of sensory perceptions compete with each other for cerebral processing capacity, and the winner of this competition is usually the physical sensation: visual mental imagery, for example, tends to be disrupted by the processing of something that one actually sees.[47] This means that we are unlikely to have an intense experience of mental imagery while we are aware of sensory stimuli coming from our physical environment, and especially while we engage consciously with them. Accordingly, in her recent book-length overview of using mental imaging in counselling and psychotherapy, Valerie Thomas states a widely accepted principle in concluding that "The everyday waking mind state is not regarded as conducive to consciously accessing the imaginal mind."[48] This is also reflected by the common experience that even when we successfully generate (or perceive) a mental image, it usually fades rapidly – the duration of the decay of the image lasts on average only a quarter of a second! – which scholars believe happens in order to avoid any disruption to physical perception.[49] In fact, even if we try consciously to exercise active maintenance of an image by mobilising attentional resources, we might be hard-pressed to hold a mental image clearly for more than a few seconds in our normal waking mind state.[50]

This being the case, the key to experiencing vivid and lasting mental imagery is to find a way of separating ourselves from the distraction of external stimuli. Experienced visualisers can achieve this by developing sufficient self-control to focus on internal stimuli so that even strong external stimuli recede from consciousness, but Samuels and Samuels are correct in asserting that for most people it is much easier to visualise if external stimuli are at a minimum.[51] Consequently, the inducement of mental imagery as a conscious application in psychology invariably takes place in specially

47 Pearson et al., "Assessing Mental Imagery," 6.
48 Thomas, *Mental Imaging in Counselling and Psychotherapy*, 76.
49 Kosslyn, Thompson and Ganis, *The Case for Mental Imagery*, 43.
50 Pearson et al., "Assessing Mental Imagery," 6.
51 Samuels and Samuels, *Seeing with the Mind's Eye*, 105.

designed environments where the interference of physical perception is reduced; a mental "quiet space" is created that allows the individual to concentrate more intensely on his/her inner state and thus to facilitate the flow of internal images. It probably does not require much justification that to have a "quiet mental space" also requires a physically quiet environment with as little noise as possible; but it may be less obvious that bright light may also hinder internal visualisation. Research has found that background luminance is an important environmental factor in this respect, as it can weaken both the generation and storage of mental imagery. This led Sherwood and Pearson to conclude that "imagery can be most effectively utilised and examined in dark environments."[52] We may add that simply closing one's eyes – as is done in so many relaxation techniques – can achieve a similar effect.

Interestingly, the intrusive nature of external stimuli has actually been made use of when trying to reduce unwanted or unbidden involuntary mental imagery. One testing area for such efforts has been the domain of dieting. It has been shown that a major contributor to food cravings is vivid sensory imagery of the appetitive target[53] – in other words, when we desire something, the image of this "something" will intrude into our minds and make the craving worse – and therefore an effective way of combating the craving is to interrupt the unwanted mental imagery. This can be accomplished by means of what is usually termed "dynamic visual noise": as Kemps and Tiggemann explain, watching, say, a flickering pattern of black and white dots can reduce the vividness of imagined objects or scenes,[54] and similarly, auditory imagery can be tackled by providing competing cognitive stimuli, for example, by counting aloud. Such application of concurrent sensory stimuli has not only been successful in interrupting or toning down desire-related mental images – and thereby suppressing various cravings (e.g. for alcohol, tobacco or food) – but also in combatting certain medical conditions such as post-traumatic stress disorder, by reducing the vividness and emotional impact of distressing memory images.[55]

Vision and altered states of consciousness

The final section of this chapter concerns the relationship of vision with various *altered states of consciousness* (ASC). These can be defined as states in which some out-of-the-ordinary content is experienced – that is, when one's sensations, perceptions, cognition and emotions are altered beyond

---

52 Sherwood and Pearson, "Closing the Mind's Eye," 4.
53 Kemps and Tiggemann, "Mental Imagery and Food Cravings," 1.
54 Ibid.; see also Baddeley and Andrade, "Working Memory and the Vividness of Imagery," 139.
55 See e.g. Kemps and Tiggemann, "Mental Imagery and Food Cravings," 1; Pearson et al., "Assessing Mental Imagery," 6.

the normal range – without displaying symptoms of any mental disorder.[56] This is, of course, a rather broad definition that subsumes a variety of mental states on a continuum between total alertness and coma,[57] but it is difficult to be more specific, because ASC are defined against a "normal" state of consciousness as a baseline, and understanding of what constitutes "normal" varies widely. Perhaps the most common characteristic of all ASC is that the individuals experiencing them recognise them as such, that is, as distinctly different from their everyday patterns of experience. However, even this criterion is somewhat fluid, because people's "everyday experiences" may also include certain enhanced states (e.g. smoking a cigarette, watching a very moving film or being in love) that can induce significant alterations in psychological functions.[58]

Similar to the faculty of vision, ASC are an integral part of human biology, which is reflected by the fact that, as Michael Winkelman concludes, "virtually all societies have practices that support the ability to function in this mode of altered consciousness."[59] This has been confirmed by a large-scale quantitative historical overview of 488 societies, in which Erika Bourguignon shows that as many as 90% of these societies utilised some form of ASC in their institutionalised social practices.[60] This high figure implies that ASC constitute a human capacity that is available universally, irrespective of historical age or sociocultural background, and what is particularly relevant to the current discussion is the fact, highlighted by Bourguignon, that "the vast majority of societies have used it . . . primarily in a sacred context."[61] Even in modern western societies, religion is one of the three main domains where ASC are discussed (with the other two being psychopathology and the drug culture).[62] These anthropological findings explain why "religious experience" is often discussed under the broad heading of ASC; for example, in his book-length overview of religious experience in early Christianity, Luke Timothy Johnson, amongst others, argues strongly against distinguishing

---

56 See e.g. Kokoszka and Wallace, "Altered States of Consciousness," 3. According to Bourguignon ("Altered States of Consciousness," 6), "altered states of consciousness are characterized by deviation in quantity of central nervous system arousal from a central, normal state." Taves (*Fits, Trances, and Vision*, 3) describes ASC as "a class of seemingly involuntary acts alternately explained in religious and secular terms. These involuntary experiences include uncontrolled bodily movements (fits, bodily exercises, falling as dead, catalepsy, convulsions); spontaneous vocalizations (crying out, shouting, speaking in tongues); unusual sensory experiences (trances, visions, voices, clairvoyance, out-of-body experiences); and alterations of consciousness and/or memory (dreams, somnium, somnambulism, mesmeric trance, mediumistic trance, hypnotism, possession, alternating personality)."
57 Robertson, *The Mind's Eye*, 27.
58 Fábián, *Altered States of Consciousness*, 5.
59 Winkelman, "Altered States of Consciousness," 24.
60 Bourguignon, "Altered States of Consciousness," 9–11.
61 Ibid., 11.
62 Ibid., 3.

"religious experiences" from the continuum of other life experiences[63] (a point we shall revisit in Chapter 5).

The three most common types of ASC typically mentioned in the literature are:

- *Various forms of relaxation and meditation.* Singer suggests that it is no accident that most psychotherapy approaches begin with some form of relaxation exercise. This helps the patient to "capture the imagery experience,"[64] that is, "to establish conditions that enhance attention to one's own ongoing imagery processes . . . [and] reduce hyperalertness to external stimulation that would blur the vividness of imagery and overload the visual system."[65] There are several techniques used to achieve a relaxed state (which some would call the "meditative zone"), but regardless of the particular process applied, it is fair to conclude that relaxation is a learnable skill in the sense that practice makes it incrementally easier and more effective. As Samuels and Samuels summarise, when people have followed a method of relaxation several times, "they may be able to relax deeply just by breathing in and out and allowing themselves to let go."[66]
- *Hypnosis.* This enigmatic state may be seen as a consciously intensified form of relaxation, in which a person, with the help of hypnotic induction rituals, is put into a hypnotic or trance state.[67]What is particularly noteworthy from our current perspective is that hypnosis relies heavily on the faculty of imagery, as reflected in the fact that a person's ability to visualise correlates positively with his/her suitability to become a subject of hypnosis.[68] In hypnosis the conscious control of the mind is inhibited and the induced trance-like state is characterised by increased suggestibility and receptivity to directions.
- *Psychoactive drug-induced states.* Drugs that impact human consciousness not only include plant-based intoxicants (e.g. cannabinoids, opioids and cocaine) or chemicals such as synthetic psychedelics (e.g. LSD), but also popular and widely used substances such as caffeine, alcohol and nicotine; indeed, the complete list of substances with some consciousness-altering capacity is very wide indeed.[69]

---

63 As Johnson (*Religious Experience*, 54) argues, "We must acknowledge at once that whatever else we say about religious experiences, they are not utterly unique but can be located among other types of experiences more or less sharing their characteristics." This view is consistent with William James's (*Varieties of Religious Experience*) influential treatment of the subject (e.g. p. 24); see also Scalise, "Visions in Jeremiah," 53–54 for a similar argument.

64 Singer, *Imagery in Psychotherapy*, 170.

65 Ibid., 171.

66 Samuels and Samuels, *Seeing with the Mind's Eye*, 110.

67 See e.g. Peter, "Hypnosis," 458–59.

68 Robertson, *The Mind's Eye*, 17.

69 See e.g. Presti, "Neurochemistry and Altered Consciousness," 24, 33.

The link between ASC and mental imagery can be partly explained on the basis of the previous discussion of our competing external and internal senses: because the everyday waking mind is less conducive to accessing mental imagery, such imagery occurs more freely under conditions in which our physical perception is suppressed. Certain altered states of consciousness can offer exactly such conditions (e.g. relaxation). Other ASC amplify mental experiences (e.g. hallucinogenic drug-induced states),[70] thereby moving the odds in the competition of the external and internal senses in favour of the latter. Irrespective of the specific method applied, however, the outcome of such altered states is an increase in the vividness and duration of visionary imagery, which means that ASC offer, in effect, optimal conditions for visualisation. This explains why visionary experiences and ASC have sometimes been treated in the literature as synonyms or as phenomena that go hand in hand, whereas, strictly speaking – as was argued earlier – this is not the case: mental imagery is a perception-like representation of an imagined reality in the brain that does not rely on the co-occurrence of any particular bodily or mental state.[71] After all, people can spend long periods of time daydreaming without reporting any signs of ASC. Having said that, it is fair to add that, just as most human activities are more fruitful in certain conditions and contexts, mental imagery burgeons within some altered states of consciousness.

Summary

The essence of this chapter is captured in a quotation from renowned Yale psychologists Jerome and Dorothy Singer, who have played a leading role in demonstrating to the scholarly community the significance and potential of vision: "Our human capacity for mental imagery representations, reenactments, and anticipatory constructions, all elaborations of our direct sensory experiences, may well be a defining characteristic of our species."[72] Vision is indeed one of the most remarkable human faculties for a number of reasons:

- The human brain is hard-wired from birth to perceive mental imagery through a built-in set of internal senses – even congenitally blind people are able to visualise to some extent.

---

70 Such amplification can be easily induced through chemical substances. Because the basic form of communication between neurons in the human brain is electro-chemical, psychoactive drugs produce chemical interaction with various molecular components of nerve cells, affecting the connection between cells. See e.g. Blätter et al., "Addiction and Altered States of Consciousness," 167; Presti, "Neurochemistry and Altered Consciousness," 24.

71 However, because of the vague definition of ASC, it is understandable that some people would consider experiencing an extensive and vivid mental image itself to be an extraordinary mental state – i.e. ASC – even if it is not accompanied by any other symptoms.

72 Singer and Singer, "Research on Imagination in Children," 11.

- This internal imagery is processed in the same neural regions as the sensory stimuli of the physical world. As a result, the brain can assign reality status to images that one sees only in the mind's eye, which means that humans can perceive vision in very much the same way that they see something real in their environment but without any external sensory input.

- In accordance with Aristotle's assertion that the "soul never thinks without a mental image," the human ability to generate and behold vision has been found to form an integral part of higher order mental functioning in general, as attested to by its central place in information processing and memory functions (both long-term and working memory).

- Psychologists consider the source of mental imagery to be previously stored information that is held in the individual's long-term or short-term memory, and which is either recalled intact or modified in creative ways. That is, from a neuropsychological perspective, mental imagery involves re-experiencing a version of stored memory images. While in the popular culture we might also find an established belief that some mental images have their sources in various external agents (e.g. spiritual forces), this belief has not been taken up or engaged with in cognitive neuroscience.

- Mental imagery involves the simulation of not only visual perception but of all the human physical senses; accordingly, people also experience auditory, tactile, olfactory and gustatory imagery. Interestingly, although visual and auditory image reports tend to be the most common, when the vividness of the imagery is ranked, the senses of smell and taste come first. A further source of variation in mental imagery concerns its purpose, which ranges from reliving memories and imagining a counterfactual scenario to picturing the future or daydreaming.

- Because of the shared neural region underlying external and internal perception, mental imagery tends to be more vivid and fades less rapidly in conditions which help to keep the distraction of external stimuli to a minimum (and thus free the processing region). Accordingly, the optimal environment for experiencing vision is one where background noise and luminance are minimal; a further facilitative condition for mental imagery is for the person involved to get into a relaxed state, as this not only suppresses external disruptions (e.g. worries or physical interferences) but also enhances attention to one's internal imagery processes.

- Vision tends to burgeon in certain human states where one's physical perception is altogether suppressed or suspended, for example in dream states during sleep or in trance-like states caused by hypnosis or various psychedelic drugs. However, we need to distinguish such altered states of consciousness from the actual perception of mental imagery, as the two phenomena concern different mental processes and do not necessarily rely on each other.

References

Baars, Bernard J. 1997. *In the Theater of Consciousness*. New York: Oxford University Press.

Baddeley, Alan D. 2003. "Working Memory and Language: An Overview." *Journal of Communication Disorders* 36: 189–208.

Baddeley, Alan D., and Jackie Andrade. 2000. "Working Memory and the Vividness of Imagery." *Journal of Experimental Psychology: General* 129, no. 1: 126–45.

Bértolo, Helder. 2005. "Visual Imagery without Visual Perception?" *Psicológica* 26: 173–88.

Blätter, Andrea E., Jörg C. Fachner, and Michael Winkelman. 2011. "Addiction and the Dynamics of Altered States of Consciousness". In *Altering Consciousness: Multidisciplinary Perspectives. Vol. 2: Biological and Psychological Perspectives*, edited by Etzel Cardeña and Michael Winkelman, 167–87. Santa Barbara, CA: Praeger.

Bourguignon, Erika. 1973. "Introduction: A Framework for the Comparative Study of Altered States of Consciousness." In *Religion, Altered States of Consciousness, and Social Change*, edited by Erika Bourguignon, 3–35. Columbus, OH: Ohio State University Press.

Brogaard, Berit, and Dimitria Electra Gatzia. 2017. "Unconscious Imagination and the Mental Imagery Debate." *Frontiers in Psychology* 8, no. 799: 1–14.

Cattaneo, Zaira, Maria Chiara Fastame, Tomaso Vecchi, and Cesare Cornoldi. 2006. "Working Memory, Imagery and Visuo-Spatial Mechanisms." In *Imagery and Spatial Cognition: Methods, Models and Cognitive Assessment*, edited by T. Vecchi and G. Bottini, 101–37. Amsterdam: John Benjamins.

Cattaneo, Zaira, and Juha Silvanto. 2015. "Mental Imagery, Psychology Of." In *International Encyclopedia of the Social and Behavioral Sciences*, edited by James Wright, 220–27. Oxford: Elsevier.

Cumming, J. L., and D. M. Ste-Marie. 2001. "The Cognitive and Motivational Effects of Imagery Training: A Matter of Perspective." *The Sport Psychologist* 15: 276–88.

Decety, Jean, and Julie Grèzes. 2006. "The Power of Simulation: Imagining One's Own and Other's Behavior." *Brain Research* 1079: 1–14.

Dewey, J. 1897. "My Pedagogic Creed". *School Journal* 54, no. 3: 77–80.

Fábián, Tibor Károly. 2012. *Mind-Body Connections: Pathways of Psychosomatic Coupling under Meditation and Other Altered States of Consciousness*. New York: Nova Science.

Fried, Itzhak, Ueli Rutishauser, Moran Cerf, and Gabriel Kreiman. 2014. *Single Neuron Studies of the Human Brain: Probing Cognition*. Cambridge, MA: MIT Press.

Gazzaniga, Michael S., Richard B. Ivry, and George R. Mangun. 2002. *Cognitive Neuroscience: The Biology of the Mind*. New York: W. W. Norton.

Hadamard, Jacques. 1945. *An Essay on the Psychology of Invention in the Mathematical Field*. Princeton, NJ: Princeton University Press.

Hall, Eric, Carol Hall, Pamela Stradling, and Diane Young. 2006. *Guided Imagery: Creative Interventions in Counselling and Psychotherapy*. London: Sage.

Horikawa, T., M. Tamaki, Y. Miyawaki, and Y. Kamitani. 2013. "Neural Decoding of Visual Imagery During Sleep." *Science* 340, no. 6132: 639–42.

James, William. 1917. *The Varieties of Religious Experience a Study in Human Nature*. New York: Longmans, Green, and Co.

Ji, Julie L., Stephanie Burnett Heyes, Colin MacLeod, and Emily A. Holmes. 2016. "Emotional Mental Imagery as Simulation of Reality: Fear and Beyond – a Tribute to Peter Lang." *Behavior Therapy* 47: 702–19.

Johnson, Luke Timothy. 1998. *Religious Experience in Earliest Christianity: A Missing Dimension in New Testament Studies*. Minneapolis, MN: Fortress.

Katz, A. N. 2000. "Mental Imagery." In *Encyclopedia of Psychology*, edited by A. E. Kazdin, 187–91. Oxford: American Psychological Association and Oxford University Press.

Kemps, Eva, and Marika Tiggemann. 2015. "A Role for Mental Imagery in the Experience and Reduction of Food Cravings." *Frontiers in Psychiatry* 5, no. 193: 1–4.

Klinger, Eric. 2009. "Daydreaming and Fantasizing: Thought Flow and Motivation." In *Handbook of Imagination and Mental Simulation*, edited by K. D. Markman, W. M. P. Klein and J. A. Suhr, 225–39. New York: Psychology Press.

Kokoszka, Andrzej, and Benjamin Wallace. 2011. "Seep, Dreams, and Other Biological Cycles as Altered States of Consciousness". In *Altering Consciousness: Multidisciplinary Perspectives. Vol. 2: Biological and Psychological Perspectives*, edited by Etzel Cardeña and Michael Winkelman, 3–20. Santa Barbara, CA: Praeger.

Kosslyn, Stephen M., John T. Cacioppo, Richard J. Davidson, Kenneth Hugdahl, William R. Lovallo, David Spiegel, and Robert Rose. 2002. "Bridging Psychology and Biology: The Analysis of Individuals in Groups." *American Psychologist* 57, no. 5: 341–51.

Kosslyn, Stephen M., and Carolyn S. Rabin. 1999. "Imagery." In *The MIT Encyclopedia of the Cognitive Sciences*, edited by R. A. Wilson and F. C. Keil, 387–89. Cambridge, MA: MIT Press.

Kosslyn, Stephen M., William L. Thompson, and Giorgio Ganis. 2006. *The Case for Mental Imagery*. New York: Oxford University Press.

Kreiman, Gabriel, Christof Koch, and Itzhak Fried. 2000. "Imagery Neurons in the Human Brain." *Nature* 408, no. 6810: 357–61.

Markus, Hazel. 2006. "Foreword." In *Possible Selves: Theory, Research and Applications*, edited by C. Dunkel and J Kerpelman, xi–xiv. New York: Nova Science.

Meister, Ingo G., Timo Krings, Henrik Foltys, Babak Boroojerdi, Mareike Müller, Rudolf Töpper, and Armin Thron. 2004. "Playing Piano in the Mind: An FMRI Study on Music Imagery and Performance in Pianists." *Cognitive Brain Research* 19: 219–28.

Modell, Arnold H. 2003. *Imagination and the Meaningful Brain*. Cambridge, MA: MIT Press.

Moulton, Samuel T., and S. M. Kosslyn. 2009. "Imagining Predictions: Mental Imagery as Mental Emulation." *Philosophical Transactions of the Royal Society B* 364: 1273–80.

Paivio, Allan. 1986. *Mental Representations: A Dual Coding Approach*. New York: Oxford University Press.

Pearson, David G., Catherine Deeprose, Sophie M. A. Wallace-Hadrill, Stephanie Burnett Heyes, and Emily A. Holmes. 2013. "Assessing Mental Imagery in Clinical Psychology: A Review of Imagery Measures and a Guiding Framework." *Clinical Psychology Review* 33: 1–23.

Pearson, Joel, and S. M. Kosslyn. 2015. "The Heterogeneity of Mental Representation: Ending the Imagery Debate." *PNAS* 112, no. 33: 10089–10092.

Pearson, Joel, Thomas Naselaris, Emily A. Holmes, and Stephen M. Kosslyn. 2015. "Mental Imagery: Functional Mechanisms and Clinical Applications." *Trends in Cognitive Sciences* 19, no. 10: 590–602.

Perkins, Pheme. 2000. "The Letter to the Ephesians: Introduction, Commentary, and Reflections." In *The New Interpreter's Bible*, edited by Leander E. Keck, 349–466. Nashville, TN: Abingdon.

Peter, Burkhard. 2015. "Hypnosis." In *International Encyclopedia of the Social and Behavioral Sciences*, edited by James Wright, 458–64. Oxford: Elsevier.

Presti, David E. 2011. "Neurochemistry and Altered Consciousness". In *Altering Consciousness: Multidisciplinary Perspectives. Vol. 2: Biological and Psychological Perspectives*, edited by Etzel Cardeña and Michael Winkelman, 21–41. Santa Barbara, CA: Praeger.

Richardson, John T. E. 1999. *Imagery*. Hove, East Sussex: Psychology Press.

Robertson, Ian. 2002. *The Mind's Eye: An Essential Guide to Boosting Your Mental Power*. London: Bantam Books.

Samuels, Mike, and Nancy Samuels. 1975. *Seeing with the Mind's Eye: The History, Techniques and Uses of Visualization*. New York: Random House.

Scalise, Pamela. 2014. "Vision Beyond the Visions in Jeremiah." In *"I Lifted My Eyes and Saw": Reading Dream and Vision Reports in the Hebrew Bible*, edited by Elizabeth R. Hayes and Lena-Sofia Tiemeyer, 47–58. London: Bloomsbury T&T Clark.

Segal, Harry G. 2006. "Possible Selves, Fantasy Distortion, and the Anticipated Life History: Exploring the Role of Imagination in Social Cognition." In *Possible Selves: Theory, Research and Applications*, edited by C. Dunkel and J Kerpelman, 79–96. New York: Nova Science.

Sherwood, Rachel, and Joel Pearson. 2010. "Closing the Mind's Eye: Incoming Luminance Signals Disrupt Visual Imagery." *PLoS One* 5, no. 12: 1–6.

Singer, Jerome L. 2006. *Imagery in Psychotherapy*. Washington, DC: American Psychological Association.

Singer, Jerome L., and Dorothy G. Singer. 2013. "Historical Overview of Research on Imagination in Children." In *The Oxford Handbook of the Development of Imagination*, edited by Marjorie Taylor, 11–27. Oxford: Oxford University Press.

Taves, Ann. 1999. *Fits, Trances, and Visions: Experiencing Religion and Explaining Experience from Wesley to James*. Princeton, NJ: Princeton University Press.

Taylor, Shelley E., Lien B. Pham, Inna D. Rivkin, and David A. Armor. 1998. "Harnessing the Imagination: Mental Simulation, Self-Regulation, and Coping." *American Psychologist* 53, no. 4: 429–39.

Thomas, Valerie. 2016. *Using Mental Imaging in Counselling and Psychotherapy: A Guide to More Inclusive Theory and Practice*. Abingdon: Routledge.

Winkelman, Michael. 2011. "A Paradigm for Understanding Altered Consciousness: The Integrative Mode of Consciousness." In *Altering Consciousness: Multidisciplinary Perspectives. Vol. 1: History, Culture, and the Humanities*, edited by Etzel Cardeña and Michael Winkelman, 23–41. Santa Barbara, CA: Praeger.

Woolfolk, Robert L., Mark W. Parrish, and Shane M. Murphy. 1985. "The Effects of Positive and Negative Imagery on Motor Skill Performance." *Cognitive Therapy and Research* 9, no. 3: 335–41.

2 Applications of vision in the social sciences

Having established the neuroscientific parameters and characteristics of vision in the previous chapter, we shall now turn to exploring how mental imagery has been utilised in various branches of psychology, sports and the business world. In doing so, we shall pay special attention to the question of what it is about vision that gives it its high motivating potential. Drawing on the intriguing theory of "possible selves" in social psychology, we will examine this question and its applications in educational contexts. Ultimately, the main goal of this chapter is to distil a number of lessons from the applied research areas reviewed that may then be helpful for an understanding of how vision can enrich and facilitate Christian life and ministry (to be discussed in the last two chapters of the book).

Vision in psychology

The study of mental imagery is currently an active and highly respected area in psychology and cognitive neuroscience. Indeed, arguably the most influential clinical psychologist to specialise in mental imagery and daydreaming, Jerome Singer, has been Professor of Psychology at the Yale School of Medicine and a former President of Division 10 of the American Psychological Association. Equally, one of the leading researchers on the neuropsychology of vision, Stephen Kosslyn, has been Head of Psychology and then Dean of Social Sciences at Harvard University. However, the subject itself has not always enjoyed such high status; as Baddeley and Andrade summarise, the study of imagery has seen "more extreme fluctuation in its scientific respectability than almost any other aspect of cognitive psychology."[1] This draws an interesting parallel with the fluctuating reputation of vision in theology (to be discussed in Chapter 6).

Although the beginning of the empirical study of vision coincides with the genesis of academic psychology at the end of the 19th century, the roots of the notion of vision can be traced back much further, even to

---

1 Baddeley and Andrade, "Working Memory and the Vividness of Imagery," 126.

Aristotle. As mentioned earlier, Aristotle considered mental imagery (*phantasma*) an integral part of human thinking, and his influential views on the link between imagery and motivation will be discussed later in some detail. The first research project on vision in the modern sense was conducted by Sir Francis Galton, who wrote an article on "Statistics of Mental Imagery"[2] in 1880, and then further discussed the subject in his book on *Inquiries into Human Faculty and Its Development.*[3] In line with his general interest in individual differences,[4] Galton's main finding on imagery was that humans differ considerably in terms of their visualisation skills, with some image reports having great vividness and clarity while others are hardly more than an outline sketch if that. We shall see later that the academic interest in imagery was also taken up by clinical psychologists (e.g. Freud and Jung) at the beginning of the 20th century, initiating a continuous tradition in psychotherapy lasting to the present day. However, in academic psychology the study of mental imagery became sidelined, if not completely banished, during the behaviourist period (roughly between the 1910s and 1960s), which placed emphasis on the experimental study of outward human behaviour rather than the introspective – and according to the behaviourists, subjective – study of human consciousness.[5] The notion of mental imagery was typically amalgamated with hallucination, which was seen as a pathological manifestation and was thus relegated to psychotherapy.[6]

   The turning point in psychological research was signalled by a paper written by Robert Holt on "Imagery: The return of the ostracized," published in the prestigious journal *American Psychologist* and based on a Presidential Address to Division 12 of the American Psychological Association that Hall delivered in 1962. He attributed this turning of the tide partly to a renewed interest shown by brain researchers and partly to the widespread appearance of psychedelic drugs and the parallel growth of psychopharmacology, which attracted a great deal of attention to imaginal phenomena in the popular press,[7] leading to bestselling publications such as *Seeing with the Mind's Eye* by Mike and Nancy Samuels.[8] There was also growing evidence that mental rehearsal could be used to improve certain motor skills,

2 Galton, "Statistics and Mental Imagery."
3 Galton, *Inquiries into Human Faculty.*
4 As Galton ("Statistics and Mental Imagery," 21) explains, "The particular branch of the inquiry to which this memoir refers, is Mental Imagery; that is to say, I desire to define the different degrees of vividness with which different persons have the faculty of recalling familiar scenes under the form of mental pictures, and the peculiarities of the mental visions of different persons."
5 For good overviews, see Thomas, *Mental Imaging in Counselling and Psychotherapy*; Curtis, "Imagery in Psychoanalysis and Psychotherapy."
6 See Holt, "Imagery," 263.
7 Ibid., 257–58, 263.
8 Samuels and Samuels, *Seeing with the Mind's Eye.*

which had considerable implications for sports performance.[9] This was also the period when humanistic psychology emerged as a major branch within the field of psychology, challenging the hegemony of behaviourism.[10] The humanistic movement introduced therapies that drew upon a wide repertoire of imagery techniques and was indirectly instrumental in unleashing a flood of literature on self-actualisation and fulfilment though visualisation techniques. As a result of all these converging trends, there was a real surge of work on images and imagination in a variety of fields, and mental imagery was reclaimed by psychology.[11]

Within psychotherapy, the healing potential of imagery was recognised right from the beginning, and was made particularly popular by Freud's and Jung's relevant work. This interest was motivated by the belief that mental imagery opens up a window into the subconscious parts of the mind and that the images and fantasies that arise can be interpreted to good effect. Freud placed high value on the analysis of dreams as sources of insight into unconscious desires, and Jung developed a technique called "active imagination," which involves free meditation with a focus on emerging images from fragments of fantasy, and even extending to engaging imagined figures in conversation.[12] After these beginnings, imagery techniques were integrated into almost all schools of psychotherapy, with cognitive behavioural therapy currently being especially known for its systematic use of mental imagery. Over the past century, several clinical innovations involving the use of various forms of visualisation have been experimented with, and some key procedures, such as guided imagery and hypnosis, have been developed and fine-tuned. In the application of vision in non-psychotherapeutic contexts (e.g. sport or education), *guided imagery* in particular plays a key role, and as such warrants a closer look.

Guided imagery

Guided imagery can be understood as controlled daydreaming, with an individual (or a group) being guided into experiencing mental images through externally provided scripts.[13] In psychotherapeutic practice, the specific form of guided imagery applied can vary on a continuum between less and more guided. At the less structured end, in one-to-one settings, the therapist or

---

9 See e.g. Feltz and Landers, "Effects of Mental Practice," 25–26.
10 E.g. Rogers, *Client-Centered Therapy*; Maslow, *Toward a Psychology of Being*.
11 As Thomas (*Mental Imaging in Counselling and Psychotherapy*, 20–21) summarises, "Faced with this evidence, behaviourists started to revise their hard-line position and began to study how imagery was implicated in behavioural change. In a very short space of time there was an explosion of interest in mental imagery. After a dearth of interest and publications, almost overnight, mental imagery was reclaimed with enthusiasm across several disciplines including psychology."
12 Ibid., 26; Hall et al., *Guided Imagery*, 12.
13 See e.g. Arbuthnott, Arbuthnott and Rossiter, "Guided Imagery."

counsellor might only suggest an opening scenario (e.g. "*Imagine a happy family occasion*") or provide an imagery theme to work with (e.g. a journey up a mountain) and then generate the imagined scenario in collaboration with the client in a dialogic format.[14] A common form of more structured guided imagery that is appropriate for group settings involves guiding people into the imaginary world by means of a *scripted scenario* that may include several suggestions and open-ended questions. The purpose is to let everybody explore their own visions, which will be unique to each person.[15] A frequent variation on this technique involves a more detailed and specific script that the participants listen to as they follow the guide's instructions in silence. This latter experience closely resembles that of reading a novel or listening to a story: the characters are described in detail, the story line is carefully delineated, and yet different individuals may still end up seeing, hearing and feeling different things because of their unique life experiences, personalities and desires.[16]

Guided imagery usually starts with a short relaxation or breathing exercise: deep, slow breathing quietens the internal organs (lowers the metabolic rate and decreases the heart rate), increases the alertness of the mind (by increasing the supply of oxygen), relaxes the participants and clears their minds of possible distractions, thereby bringing about the appropriate emotional climate for images to readily appear. An extension of deep relaxation is the "positive imagery approach," whereby after one's mind has been cleared, the individual is encouraged to think of a pleasant memory or scene (usually a nature scene) and to visualise it in as much detail and clarity as possible. The goal is, as Seymour Epstein explains, that one should keep coming back to the same scene and work on it until it can be called up at a moment's notice – five minutes a day for about a month is usually enough to gain sufficient proficiency in doing so.[17] Imagining such highly pleasurable and relaxing scenes has been found to be effective in counteracting anxiety, and the practice of consciously pairing such internal pictures with anxiety-arousing images is an established method of systematic

14 See e.g. Hall et al., *Guided Imagery*, 57.
15 An example adapted from Dörnyei and Kubanyiova (*Motivating Learners*, 49): "Imagine yourself with friends . . . where are you? . . . what does the place look like? . . . what can you see around you? . . . how many people are there? . . . what do they look like? . . . what are they wearing? . . . what can you hear? . . . what are you doing? . . . what are you wearing? . . . you are speaking to someone . . . who is it? . . . what do they look like? . . . what are you talking about? . . . how do people react to you? . . . etc."
16 An example adapted from Arbuthnott et al. ("Guided Imagery," 123): "Imagine that you are walking across a field of fresh green grass on a warm spring day. You feel the softness of the grass beneath your feet, the warmth of the air on your skin, and hear the sound of birds singing in the distance. You are moving toward a large tree that is near a creek. When you reach the tree, you sit down with your back supported by the trunk. Listening to the soft sound of running water in the creek, you notice that you are filled with a sense of well-being ."
17 Epstein, *Constructive Thinking*, 231.

desensitization treatment of phobias (i.e. a managed incremental exposure to the phobic target, offset by intensive relaxation).[18]

Transportation theory

Guided imagery has been found to serve as an effective tool for inducing mental imagery in the listeners, but our account would not be complete without the discussion of a related form of capturing the imagination, the intriguing psychological theory of *transportation*.[19] This theory grew out of the recognition of the distinctive power of stories and narrative worlds, and its primary focus is on *transportation experience*, that is, exploring the human condition of becoming so immersed in a story that people temporarily leave their own realities behind. This is the experience we have when, for example, we are engrossed in reading a real page-turner, or when we can sit watching an exciting "box set" for hours and hours. Indeed, it is the transportation power of biblical narratives that has been a key factor in the birth of narrative theology.[20] Green and Donahue explain what is involved in a true transportation experience as follows:

> Imagine a person immersed in a favourite mystery novel. This person may not hear others enter or leave a room while she is reading. She may stay up late into the night because she does not realise how much time has gone by. Her heart may start beating faster during tense moments in the plot, or she may laugh or cry along with the main characters in the story. She may have a vivid mental image of the appearance of these characters.[21]

Listening to stories and following their narrative trails can be an imaginative and immersive experience, similar to other forms of mental simulation,[22] and thus it can be used effectively to facilitate the evoking and strengthening of visions: according to the Transportation-Imagery Model,[23] compelling narratives create transportation experience, which, in turn, generates mental imagery in the reader/listener, making them feel as if they were experiencing the events themselves. The transportation experience links these images with the beliefs or new perspectives contained in the story, which explains the potency of narrative-based persuasion.

18 Singer, *Imagery in Psychotherapy*, 111; Thomas, *Mental Imaging in Counselling and Psychotherapy*, 36.
19 Green and Brock, "The Role of Transportation"; see Green and Donahue, "Simulated Worlds" for a recent review.
20 See e.g. Crites, "The Narrative Quality of Experience"; for a review, see Dörnyei, *Progressive Creation*, 5–12.
21 Green and Donahue, "Simulated Worlds," 241.
22 Ibid., 243.
23 Ibid., 245.

Vision and performance in sport

In professional sports the stakes are high, and therefore a great deal of research has been conducted on how mental imagery can be used to facilitate performance. On balance, studies have found that imagery is effective in promoting achievement.[24] As a result, virtually every elite athlete in the world applies some sort of imagery enhancement technique during training.[25] In fact, it has been found that imagery training is the most widely applied psychological skills training technique among both athletes and coaches/sport psychologists.[26]

Interestingly, as Munroe-Chandler and Guerrero's review highlights, most of the recent research on sport performance has been based on an analytic model developed by Allan Paivio, the same author of dual coding theory described earlier.[27] Because this is arguably the most useful model in the literature to summarise the various roles that imagery can play in human performance, and some of its tenets will also be relevant to facilitating Christian life, let us take a closer look. The strength of Paivio's model is that it brings together a number of different imagery functions employed in sports along two central dimensions: *cognitive* and *motivational*. The former involves imagery used by athletes for mental rehearsal in order to plan, refine and practise various strategies, routines and specific motor skills (e.g. as mentioned earlier, putting in golf); the latter, the motivational functions, are those that pertain to bigger picture goals, such as visualising winning a gold medal at the Olympics, thereby helping to keep the athletes' commitment at a high level. In essence, as Richard Cox summarises, an athlete can use imagery "to plan a winning strategy (cognitive function) or to get energised for competition (motivational function)."[28] Paivio further divided these two main dimensions, cognitive and motivational, into two subcategories, general and specific, and then Hall, Mack, Paivio and Hausenblas extended the motivational general function to include two subtypes,[29] thus resulting in the following five-component framework:

1. *Cognitive General* function: using mental imagery to familiarise oneself with the competition site or to rehearse team strategies and entire game plans (e.g. set pieces in football such as a corner kick).

---

24 See e.g. Gregg and Hall, "Motivational Imagery in Sport," 961.
25 Weinberg and Gould (*Sport and Exercise Psychology*, 298) report that in a study conducted at the United States Olympic Training Center, 90% of Olympic athletes used some form of imagery and that 91% of them considered this practice useful. The proportion of coaches using imagery training was even higher: 94%, with one-fifth applying imagery at every training session.
26 Morris, "Imagery," 481.
27 Munroe-Chandler and Guerrero, "Imagery in Sport," 1–2.
28 Cox, *Sport Psychology*, 277.
29 Hall, Mack, Paivio and Hausenblas, "Imagery Use by Athletes."

2. *Cognitive Specific* function: imaging oneself correctly executing a specific sport skill (e.g. a basketball free throw).
3. *Motivational General – Arousal* function: imagery associated with managing stress or arousal associated with performing (e.g. relaxing or psyching up).
4. *Motivational General – Mastery* function: imagining oneself in a situation exhibiting the ability to remain mentally tough, focused and confident (e.g. coping in an important competition or remaining positive in the face of a tough challenge or previous disappointment).
5. *Motivational Specific* function: imaging oneself in a highly motivating situation, accomplishing an individual goal (e.g. scoring the winning point in the national championship, achieving a personal best time or stepping onto the podium to receive a gold medal).

The imagery involved in these functions might include both recalling peak achievements or past success (e.g. beating a formidable competitor) or, alternatively, forming creative images about a successful future performance. These images can be used to reduce negative thoughts by focusing on a positive outcome and also to build confidence, increase concentration and maintain momentum, for example, during injury.[30] They can help athletes to "up their game" when training becomes sluggish. Finally, they can offer a mental run through the complete performance (e.g. in diving), thereby setting the stage, and even giving the athlete the opportunity to practice mentally correcting mistakes before the real performance. It has also been shown that visual and audio input can be used to develop constructive imagery skills. In a volume on sport psychology published by the American Psychological Association, Gould, Damarjian and Greenleaf explain that "success tapes," which contain some of the athletes' best competition moments or some edited, "perfect" performances, can have a strong motivational effect: "For example, the 1998 U.S. women's ice hockey team used an imagery tape of season highlights interspersed with Muhammad Ali clips to create positive feelings of confidence before their gold medal-winning game."[31] The researchers added that the athletes' favourite music can be "dubbed onto the tape to serve as a cue to trigger excellent performance in the future", and listening to this music on a portable stereo headset can be helpful to trigger

---

30 Having successfully returned to the top after a serious injury by winning the Australian open in 2019, tennis star Novak Djokovic said the following at a press conference: "I think probably the biggest secret of my success, if I can say, or probably any other athlete, is self-belief. Always digging deep in the moments when you're facing adversity, digging those moments of complimenting yourself, visualising yourself as a winner, trying to be in a positive state of mind." (www.bbc.co.uk/sport/tennis/47021517) I am grateful to Norbert Schmitt for drawing my attention to this quote.
31 Gould, Damarjian and Greenleaf, "Imagery Training," 65.

feelings of success in situations in which it is not practical to watch a vide-otape (e.g. at a competitive venue).[32]

Let us conclude this section with what many would probably consider to be the most astonishing impact of imagery in sport, namely the fact that not only can visualisation improve the precision of certain skills but it can also contribute to actual muscle gain. That is, in theory, we can increase our physical strength through mental imagery without going to the gym! The neuroscientific basis of this remarkable finding is that by going through a training routine mentally, many of the same brain circuits will be activated – and thus strengthened and fine-tuned – as if one participated in the activity with one's physical body; the brain signals, in turn, drive the muscles to a higher activation level and thus increase their strength.[33] According to a recent review by Slimani and his colleagues, laboratory studies have consist-ently evidenced measurable strength gain as a result of mental imagery.[34] For example, in a 12-week training programme (15 minutes per day, 5 days per week), consisting purely of visualisation without performing any physi-cal exercises, a 13.5% muscle strength increase was observed,[35] while in a similar study lasting for 6 weeks the gain was 10.8%.[36] In another study that involved mixing physical and mental practice in four training exer-cises (bench press, leg press, triceps extension and calf raise), the researchers found that replacing some of their physical training routines with mental imagery did not cause any significant performance reduction.[37]

---

32 Ibid.
33 Robertson, *The Mind's Eye*, 203; Ranganathan et al., "From Mental Power to Muscle Power," 944.
34 Slimani et al., "Effects of Mental Imagery on Muscular Strength," 434.
35 Ranganathan et al., "From Mental Power to Muscle Power," 944.
36 Yao et al., "Kinesthetic Imagery Training," 1.
37 Reiser, Büsch and Munzert, "Motor Imagery," 6. The question, though, is why one should replace physical exercise with mental ones, given that it is arguably harder and less fun to practice mental imagery than to work out or play a sport. Research has come up with two responses: first, in one study (Lebon, Collet and Guillot, "Motor Imagery training," 1680), two groups were asked to do regular bench press and leg press exercises, but when they took a break from the physical exercise, one of the groups was instructed to carry on the task mentally (while physically resting). The extra mental exercise was shown to have paid off in added strength, indicating that training can be intensified by utilising physical rest periods for mental practice. Perhaps more importantly, other studies showed that mental training can also take place when an athlete would be prevented from physical training because of a sports injury. For example, in one study, two groups of healthy participants underwent wrist-hand immobilisation – they were fitted with a rigid cast extending from just below the elbow past the fingers – to induce a temporary weakness in their wrist. Over a period of four weeks in cast, as expected, a 45% loss of strength occurred, but signifi-cantly, in those subjects who regularly exercised their wrists mentally, the loss of strength was reduced by as much as 50% (Clark et al., "Power of the Mind," 3222; similar results were obtained by Meugnot and Agbangla, "Motor Imagery Practice," 496). This means

Vision and business management

As in psychology and sports, we find frequent uses of the term "vision" in the business world, albeit used in a slightly different way and with a meaning that does not fully coincide with that of "mental imagery" that we have discussed earlier. Rather than referring to an internal image, "vision in business" tends to be used in close association, and sometimes even interchangeably, with terms such as "goal" (e.g. *"the company's goal/vision is to become the market leader"*) or "mission" (e.g. *"the organisation's vision/ mission statement"*), and at some other times it is used in an even broader sense, referring to the values, strategies and the philosophy underlying an organisation or venture (e.g. *"our vision is a workplace that promotes individual creativity"*).[38] We saw in the previous chapter that the main difference between a vision proper and a mission/goal lies in the pictorial detail that a vision comprises. Despite the somewhat inconsistent usages of the term "vision" in the world of business (and politics), the various meanings all contain elements of an imagined ideal future state. For example, in their highly influential seminal book on leadership – which is already on its sixth edition and has sold over two million copies in over 20 languages since its original publication in 1987 – James Kouzes and Barry Posner defined vision as "an ideal and unique image of the future,"[39] and variations on this definition are included in most relevant works in the business management literature.[40] While this conception is fully compatible with previous discussions of mental imagery, Kouzes and Posner go one step further when they describe vision in the corporate world as follows:

> Visions are images of the mind; they are impressions and representations. They become real as leaders express those images in concrete terms to their constituents. Just as architects make drawings and engineers build models, leaders find ways of giving expression to collective hopes for the future. . . . Vision statements, then, are not statements at all. They are pictures – word pictures. They are images of the future. For people to share a vision, they have to see it in their mind's eye.[41]

This understanding extends the meaning of vision in an important way. While in psychology the focus of mental imagery is on how imagined reality

---

that athletes who temporarily cannot participate in a conventional fitness programme can still improve their motor functions through engaging with mental practice.

38 E.g. Collins and Porras ("Company Vision," 66) conclude, "But vision has become one of the most overused and least understood words in the language, conjuring up different images for different people: of deeply held values, outstanding achievement, societal bonds, exhilarating goals, motivating forces, or raisons d'être."

39 Kouzes and Posner, *The Leadership Challenge*, 97.

40 See e.g. Berg, "Purpose and Goals in Visions," 3; Strange and Mumford, "Origins of Vision," 344.

41 Kouzes and Posner, *The Leadership Challenge*, 132.

is represented mentally, vision in business also involves some form of wider *sharing* with an audience for a purpose; as Kouzes and Posner put it in the prior quotation, visions "become real as leaders express those images in concrete terms to their constituents." Levin also argues that vision is not simply a destination to seek but "a field that permeates the entire organization, affecting all who bump up against it."[42] In other words, while mental imagery is usually a private experience for an individual, a business leader's personal vision serves only as the initial seed that will need to grow into a corporate or collective vision in order to empower the people involved in the business. This has two important implications:

(a) Although a successful business vision typically has at its core some mental imagery perceived by an originator (often, but not necessarily the leader), this initial imagery is then elaborated on – often with the help of others – into an *expanded canvas* to be appropriated by a whole community. As Levin puts it, an organisational vision is "a highly lucid story of an organization's preferred future in action. A future that describes what life will be like for employees, customers, and other key stakeholders."[43]

(b) Given that a vision needs to be shared in order to become successful, the way in which that initial vision is described assumes crucial importance. In other words, the quality of the *vision report* (or as it is usually termed in business circles, the "vision statement") will matter very much. The recurring advice in the business literature is that the vision statement should contain *image-based rhetoric*, as this can evoke a mental picture in the followers, which in turn can be the foundation for their own personal visions.[44] In this sense, a vision statement can serve as the script of guided imagery for others. We shall see in the next chapter that while the term "vision" in the Bible is typically reserved for individual mental imagery in a psychological sense, some of the vision reports recorded in the Scriptures (e.g. Moses's description of the Promised Land) share similarities with corporate vision statements in that they are carefully crafted and in some cases are expressed in elaborate details.

Thus, vision in the business sense is similar to mental imagery in psychology in terms of its pictorial quality, but it tends to be described in expressive language and it also has a prominent motivational dimension, because its primary purpose is to provide the members of an organisation with a sense of purpose, direction and impetus. Let us look more closely at the qualities of an effective vision statement before examining the inherent motivational capacity of vision.

---

42 Levin, "Vision Revisited," 103.
43 Ibid., 93.
44 Stam, van Knippenberg and Wisse, "Focusing on Followers," 458.

The quality of the vision statement

Broadly speaking, while the focus of the discussion of vision in psychology is on the qualities of the internal experience, the emphasis in the corporate world is on the potential impact of the vision shared with others. Therefore, the overall quality of a vision in business depends rather less on the clarity and vividness of the original mental representation of the envisioned reality and more on the clarity and vividness of the vision statement formed as a result of that initial representation. After all, a vision's worth in business terms is measured by the degree to which people desire to embrace it. We saw in the previous chapter Ira Levin's detailed description of what constitutes a good vision statement, namely that the vision should be "so vivid as to enable the listener or reader to transport himself or herself to the future, so to speak, to witness it and experience it."[45] An example of how this can be done is in Henry Ford's description of his vision of a world of cars, spoken at a time when horses were the dominant engines of the highways:

> I will build a motor car for the great multitude. . . . It will be so low in price that no man making a good salary will be unable to own one and enjoy with his family the blessing of hours of pleasure in God's great open spaces. . . . When I'm through, everybody will be able to afford one, and everyone will have one. The horse will have disappeared from our highways, the automobile will be taken for granted . . . [and we will] give a large number of men employment at good wages.[46]

In contrast, ineffective mission statements, according to Collins and Porras, are "usually a boring, confusing, structurally unsound stream of words that evoke the response 'True, but who cares?' "[47] It is in "who cares?" that the real problem lies, because a business vision that people cannot see is indeed pointless. In the light of this, what are the attributes of a truly effective vision statement? Here is a list of some key elements:

- *Vivid description of a better place.* For the shared vision to make an impact, it needs to involve a vibrant, engaging and specific portrayal of what it will be like to achieve the desired target. It goes without saying that the image will only be attractive if it represents a better place than where the beholders currently are.
- *Enthusiasm and excitement.* Enthusiasm is infectious and excitement can ignite the same passion in others. These qualities need to shine through the vision statement to convince the receivers that the proposal is worthy of their time and support.[48] Or, to look at it from the other

45 Levin, "Vision Revisited," 95.
46 Cited in Collins and Porras, "Company Vision," 74.
47 Ibid., 76.
48 Kouzes and Posner, *The Leadership Challenge*, 16.

perspective, if the sharers of the vision cannot display enthusiasm and excitement for their own proposal, the receivers will quickly get the message that there is nothing there to get excited about.

- *Inclusive nature.* Stam and his colleagues rightly point out that visions which invite the beholders to imagine themselves as a positive part of the future are particularly motivating; in such cases, "the image may be personalized into an ideal future self-image for followers."[49] (The question of ideal self-images will be discussed further in a separate section later.) Kouzes and Posner put it this way: "You have to *show them* how to realise *their* dreams. . . . You have to make the connection between an inspiring vision of the future and the personal aspirations and passions of the people you are addressing."[50] Thus, a key feature of an effective vision is that it is inclusive and that it motivates people to join the campaign and add their own worth.

- *Core ideology.* In their seminal paper on company vision in the *Harvard Business Review*, Collins and Porras argue that besides a description of the envisioned future, a well-conceived vision should also contain a component that they labelled as "core ideology," which defines "the enduring character of an organization."[51] They describe "enduring character" as consisting of more than merely core values and core purpose, but rather touching upon the fundamental "culture," "flavour" or "essence" of the organisation – hence, "core ideology." This almost sensual quality is what adds value to a "brand" – a key term in the contemporary business world – and as we shall see in Chapter 6, the quality of the culture will also be highly relevant to the vision of churches and church organisations.

- *Clear finish line.* Collins and Porter are right in stating that "people like to shoot for finish lines,"[52] that is, a specific end goal, which allows the whole organisation to know when they have achieved the objective. In contemporary language, this finish line is often referred to as a "target."

Vision and human motivation

The previous overview of the application of vision in business management and leadership studies has highlighted a fundamental feature of vision, its ability to *motivate*; Kurland and her colleagues offer a concise summary of this motivational dimension:

> However, vision is more than an image of the future. It has the power to inspire, motivate, and engage people. Vision rallies people for a joint effort, motivates them to become involved and committed, promoting

49 Stam et al., "Focusing on Followers," 457.
50 Kouzes and Posner, *The Leadership Challenge*, 127.
51 Collins and Porras, "Company Vision," 66.
52 Ibid., 73.

quality performance, causing them to exert additional efforts and
devote time. . . .[53]

We have seen that the notion of vision has also been used in sports to motivate athletes and to enhance performance, and given that vision in the most
general sense is a "statement for a transformation"[54] (van der Helm), it is fair
to conclude that the term has an inherent motivational connotation. Indeed,
if someone claims to have a vision, we would rightly expect that person to
pursue it (and not doing so would be considered odd). Organisational visions
are also drawn up with the explicit purpose of guiding and energising – that
is, motivating – the members' activity or work. Therefore, we can say that
the act of conjuring up internal pictures has strong motivational potential.[55]

Curiously, while there is general agreement amongst scholars about the
motivational dimension of envisioned future pictures or plans, there is
less certainty about the specific mechanisms that mediate the motivational
impact of such mental imagery. The quote from Kurland and her colleagues
cited earlier is fairly typical in this respect in that the motivational impact
of vision is taken for granted and is simply declared rather than explained.
Such claims beg the question of *why* a mental image of a future scenario
would be instrumental in realising a desired outcome; or, in van der Helm's
words, "How can a bunch of ideas depicting an idealised future provoke
and sustain behaviour, which tends to strive for this particular future?"[56]
The following overview will demonstrate that despite the absence of a definite answer to this question, there has been no scarcity of relevant reflection
and research; to the contrary: there have been several proposals in psychology aiming to justify why and how vision can motivate behaviour.

Psychological theories of the link between vision and motivation

In 1998, four psychologists from UCLA published an influential paper
in *American Psychologist*, the official academic journal of the American

53 Kurland, Peretz and Hertz-Lazarowitz, "Leadership Style," 13.
54 van der Helm, "The Vision Phenomenon," 102.
55 One may argue in this respect that the motivational dimension of vision is only relevant
    when the term concerns an imagined *future* state – as it usually does in the business world –
    whereas we saw in the previous chapter that the notion of mental imagery also subsumes
    recalling past experiences (i.e. memory images) or fantasising about "what would have
    happened if . . .?" (i.e. counterfactual thinking). While it is true that the motivational
    impact of vision is typically discussed in the literature with regard to envisioned *future*
    scenarios, it is important to note that autobiographical memories have also been found to
    serve directive functions in that they inform, guide and inspire the person who remembers
    (see e.g. Pillemer, "Autobiographical Memory," 193), and counterfactual fantasies have
    been seen to have a similar functional impact on behavioural intentions and motivation (see
    e.g. Epstude and Roese, "Counterfactual Thinking," 168).
56 van der Helm, "The Vision Phenomenon," 101.

Psychological Association, focusing on "Harnessing the Imagination." As a starting point, Shelley Taylor and her colleagues asserted that "Of the many skills that humans possess, one of the most intriguing is the process by which we envision the future and then regulate our behaviour and emotions so as to bring it about."[57] The human faculty to imagine future events, they explain, has been explored in virtually every area of psychology, from *developmental psychology* (e.g. examining how children fantasise and make plans) and *cognitive psychology* (e.g. studying how people deploy mental resources to manage vision-related tasks) to *personality* and *social psychology* (e.g. exploring how people's envisioning of themselves in the future can guide their self-concepts and actions), and last but not least, *clinical psychology* (e.g. helping clients to rehearse coping skills in their minds in order to manage potentially problematic future situations). If we add to this spectrum the interest in the neural processes underlying mental imagery in *cognitive neuroscience* as well as the copious applications of visualisation in the worlds of *sports* and *business*, we may agree with Taylor and her colleagues that the capacity to generate, behold and manipulate visions of the future is indeed a most impressive and intriguing human skill, linked to a wide range of possible research perspectives and applications.

The different approaches to understanding how vision is related to motivated behaviour have produced a range of theoretical explanations. From these it appears that the motivational capacity of vision can be explained by the fact that it can trigger off a number of different mechanisms. This ensures that most people will be positively affected by at least some of the activated processes – to put it broadly, vision can stir up something in virtually everybody. For our current discussion, three theoretical issues in particular are relevant: (a) possible selves theory; (b) the link between vision and emotions; and (c) vision as a behavioural compass.

Possible future selves

Arguably the most elaborate psychological explanation for the motivational capacity of vision has been offered by the theory of *possible selves*[58] and especially the study of the *ideal* and *ought selves*.[59] "Possible selves" are people's ideas of what they *might* become, what they *would like* to become or even what they are *afraid of* becoming in the future; in Oyserman and James' words, they are:

> the future-oriented aspects of self-concept, the positive and negative selves that one expects to become or hopes to avoid becoming. They are

57 Taylor et al., "Harnessing the Imagination," 429.
58 Markus and Nurius, "Possible Selves"; for a review, see Dunkel and Kerpelman, *Possible Selves*.
59 Higgins, "Self-Discrepancy."

the desired and feared images of the self already in a future state – the 'clever' self who passed the algebra test, the 'unhealthy' self who failed to lose weight or quit smoking, and the 'off-track' self who became pregnant. Individuals possess multiple positive and negative possible selves.[60]

Significantly from our current perspective, possible selves have been conceptualised not as abstract notions but as *pictures* of oneself through *mental imagery*. The chief proponents of the theory, Hazel Markus and Paula Nurius, emphasised that possible selves are represented in the mind in the same imaginary and semantic way as the here-and-now self[61] – that is, they can feel like reality for the individual: people can see and hear their possible future selves. This understanding makes possible selves similar to visions about oneself, and indeed, Markus and Nurius confirm that "Possible selves encompass within their scope visions of desired and undesired end states."[62] Thus, possible selves can be seen as the "vision of what might be."[63]

The *ideal self* is one key type of these potential future selves, representing a desired "best-case" scenario (i.e. the best that one can conceivably be), for example becoming a successful business tycoon or, to take a more spiritual angle, an effective missionary with a wide sphere of influence. Thus, the ideal self represents a person's own internal desires, which is in contrast to another image, the *ought self*, which represents other people's (e.g. friends' or parents') visions for that person, for example when a parent projects onto their child the image of becoming a successful doctor. This is therefore an "imported" image which reflects the attributes that one believes one ought to possess to meet expectations and to avoid possible negative outcomes. The ideal and the ought selves have been found to play a decisive role in shaping people's actions.[64]

How can an image of oneself in the future exert any motivational force in the present? The most common explanation of this force has drawn on *self-discrepancy theory*,[65] arguing that a perceived discrepancy between actual and desired selves creates an unease in the person about the difference and thus generates an urge to reduce the gap by making efforts to approach the desired self. Other scholars have considered desired future self-images to be *incentives* for future behaviour (thus having a "pulling power") or *behavioural standards* to reconcile one's behaviour with[66] (thus having a normative power), while still others have emphasised the *hope* associated with

60 Oyserman and James, "Possible Selves," 373.
61 Markus and Nurius, "Possible Selves," 961.
62 Markus and Nurius, "Motivation and the Self-Concept," 159.
63 Ibid.
64 See e.g. Dörnyei, "Future Self-Guides and Vision," 12, for a summary of how this works in the field of language education.
65 Higgins, "Self-Discrepancy," 154.
66 Hoyle and Sherrill, "Future Orientation," 1687.

a visualised future state as the main driver of action.[67] While different in their emphasis, all these view motivation "as a reflection of what individuals hope to accomplish with their life and the kind of people they would like to become,"[68] and converge upon the tenet that the pursuit of a sought-after self-image will energise action.

Vision and emotions

In mental imagery, individuals mentally mimic not only sensory images and motor movements but also *emotional experiences*. Indeed, imagining a scenario can evoke an emotional state that is as powerful as physically experiencing the same scenario. For example, the main symptoms of post-traumatic stress disorder (PTSD) are the powerful disruptive emotions that are produced by imagery in the form of 'flashbacks' to the original traumatic event.[69] While there is no question that emotions can considerably shape human behaviour, and thus possess motivational power, curiously, psychology has typically treated the two concepts of emotion and motivation separately, without focusing on the connection between them.[70] In their seminal paper, Taylor and her colleagues acknowledged that envisaging an outcome may be effective in engaging an emotional response that in turn can help people to muster the motivation to achieve their goals. However, they also highlight the fact that emotional arousal in itself, without a suitable action plan, does not guarantee productive goal-appropriate behaviour[71] (e.g. being excited about something does not necessarily lead to being productive). This might be related to Silvan Tomkins's classic observation on emotions, namely that their main impact involves *amplifying* human reactions and responses without necessarily giving them direction.[72] In order to provide specific direction for action, some kind of additional cognitive process needs to be involved, and experts are divided on what this process entails.[73] (The necessary conditions for action will be discussed in the next section.)

---

67 Boyatzis and Akrivou, "The Ideal Self," 626.
68 Leondari, Syngollitou and Kiosseoglou, "Future Selves," 154.
69 Holmes and Matthews, "Mental Imagery in Emotion," 350.
70 E.g. Reeve's classic volume on *Understanding Motivation and Emotion*, which is now on its sixth edition, discusses the two concepts relatively unconnectedly, without any explicit focus on the emotional basis of motivation.
71 Taylor et al., "Harnessing the Imagination," 432.
72 As Tomkins (*Affect, Imagery, Consciousness*, 659) summarises, "Affect amplifies, in an abstract way, any stimulus which evokes it or any response which it may recruit and prompt, be the response cognitive or motoric. Thus, an angry response usually has the abstract quality of the high-level neural firing of anger, no matter what its more specific qualities in speech or action. An excited response is accelerating in speed whether in walking or talking. An enjoyable response is decelerating in speed and relaxed as a motor or perceptual savouring response."
73 For an insightful review, see Baumeister et al., "How Emotion Shapes Behavior."

There are two further aspects of the emotional content of vision that are worthy of note here, as they can have a bearing on motivation. First, because mental imagery evokes emotional responses, it can enable people to "try out" the emotional consequences of certain behaviours,[74] for example by imagining how they would feel in a specific situation. This, in turn, allows them to carry out certain emotional "cost-benefit calculations," the outcome of which will inevitably influence their motivation and future action. Indeed, as Roy Baumeister and his colleagues conclude in a review article, "anticipated emotion may be more important in guiding behaviour than actual, felt emotion."[75] Second, on the basis of the close correspondence between emotional impulses in real and imaged situations, it is possible to use carefully crafted visual stimuli to create in people positive emotional responses to achievement situations, thereby increasing their psychological willingness to expose themselves to such stimuli in the real world. A good example of this would be the practice of using "success tapes" in sport (mentioned earlier), which contain some of the athletes' best competition moments or some edited, perfect performances.

The link between emotions, vision and motivated behaviour is arguably at its strongest when it comes to negative affect, especially *fear*: we all know that the determination to avoid an undesirable life situation can be a powerful motive. Researchers have found that hoped-for outcomes will have a stronger motivational impact if the person also bears in mind the "other side of the coin," that is, the negative situation that could arise if the desired state was *not* realised.[76] Moreover, the fear evoked by mental imagery can also be utilised to positive effect in clinical treatment of people. It was mentioned earlier that psychotherapy has traditionally employed imagery for the systematic desensitisation of people with phobias through exposing them incrementally to a phobic target. This "getting-used-to" function can be applied more broadly: there is a solid body of research showing that mental imagery can be harnessed for "fear-extinction learning," that is, learning and rehearsing new emotional responses to help people to face and engage with stressful situations that they would have steered clear of and avoided in the past.[77]

Vision as a behavioural compass

The belief that vision has the potency to direct action can be traced back to Aristotle, who defined the image in the soul as the prime motivating force in human behaviour and one which also acts as a behavioural guide.[78] Yet,

74 Ji et al., "Emotional Mental Imagery," 703–704.
75 Baumeister et al., "How Emotion Shapes Behavior," 190.
76 See e.g. Markus and Ruvolo, "Possible Selves," 223.
77 Ji et al., "Emotional Mental Imagery," 703.
78 For a review, see McMahon, "Images as Motives," 465.

it was also mentioned that the exact nature of this latter point – that is, *how* vision works as a behavioural compass – has been ambiguous, with some scholars claiming that *outcome simulation* (i.e. focusing exclusively on the outcome to be achieved) is insufficient without effectively planning the route to the imagined target.[79] They would argue that without envisioning the specific steps involved in reaching a goal – that is, without adopting a *process focus* – the imagery will not be powerful enough to lead to increased performance.[80] However, we must not dismiss the power of an outcome focus altogether: an elaborate future scenario entertained by someone in their mind's eye can have a directive function through causing a deep sense of *satisfaction* when that person's actions/decisions are aligned with the future vision.[81] Dörnyei, Henry and Muir describe this self-satisfaction as follows:

> it is a feeling of being in a state of harmony, of doing something that is personally rewarding, and which connects with an individual's true sense of *who they really are* and where they are going in life . . . a base core of *connectedness* between activity and identity. . . .[82]

In a sense, the "jury is still out" regarding the extent to which a vision can provide specific direction (rather than merely general orientation), and this is well reflected in the rather cautious statement from the initiators of possible selves theory, Markus and Nurius: "*Very often* [future self-images] also include some idea about the ways to achieve these ends"[83] (emphasis added). This is probably a realistic assessment: elaborate future visions undoubtedly function as *magnets* whose attractive force pulls people towards the desired goal, but they also have certain qualities of a *compass* in that they outline, or point to, some aspects of a course of action towards this goal.

The promotion of vision

To conclude this overview of the scientific literature on mental imagery, we shall consider strategies that have been developed to enable people to access their capability to visualise and to intensify this experience. One may rightly ask at this point why such strategies are necessary, given that vision has been described earlier as a universally recognised, hard-wired human faculty that everybody is assumed to possess. While this is true, it does not follow that everybody can use this faculty equally effectively, and indeed, we find

---

79 Taylor et al., "Harnessing the Imagination," 438.
80 Ibid.; see also Vasquez and Buehler, "Seeing Future Success," 1393.
81 See e.g. Boyatzis and Akrivou, "The Ideal Self," 626.
82 Dörnyei, Henry and Muir, *Motivational Currents*, 103.
83 Markus and Nurius, "Motivation and the Self-Concept," 159.

considerable individual differences in people's ability to employ visualisation.[84] As we shall see, these differences can occur for a variety of reasons, and the sections below will describe some established approaches both to increasing the effectiveness of people's visualisation skills and to alleviating some of the underlying problems that may hold some back.

A second and related area concerns the inconsistent motivational impact of mental simulation itself. It has been observed that some envisaged future scenarios are more inspiring than others, and that sometimes even the most vividly detailed future image fails to elicit relevant action. Research has found that this variation arises from the fact that in order for a desired image of the future to exert its energising capacity, some *essential conditions* need to be in place. Therefore, it will be useful to identify in what follows some of the key characteristics that enable the transference of mental imagery into motivated action.

Enhancing imagery skills

Singer, amongst others, observes that when asked, many people report little or no capacity for generating vivid mental images.[85] Why should this be? Singer suggests that such problems with producing imagery may often be traceable to insufficient childhood experiences with pretend play,[86] leaving the faculty of vision in effect yet to be unlocked. On the other hand, as we have seen earlier, mental imagery is also part of everyday cognitive operations (e.g. memory functions), which means that virtually everybody will be able to recall the image of, say, an apple or the colour of the wallpaper in their bedroom. In fact, Epstein is right to point out that in many cases when people think they cannot visualise, it is because they assume this to involve conjuring up mental images as clear as those in a photograph or a movie; whereas, as Epstein explains, most people most of the time visualise vague and general impressions of things.[87] Related to this point, Singer emphasises that people's attitudes towards visualisation can also affect the process itself;[88] broadly speaking, someone who attaches more significance to the role of visualisation is likely to perceive more elaborate imagery than someone who considers this a frivolous and superficial daydreaming exercise. Likewise, a person who is willing to scaffold the imaginative process by applying initial relaxation techniques is more likely to have better results than people who do not consider such preparation to be necessary. All this

---

84 This was in fact the subject of the first-ever scientific study on vision in psychology by Galton ("Statistics of Mental Imagery").
85 Singer, *Imagery in Psychotherapy*, 117.
86 Ibid., 169.
87 Epstein, *Constructive Thinking*, 242.
88 Singer, *Imagery in Psychotherapy*, 173.

points to the conclusion that very often *the vividness of a picture is in the (mind's) eye of the beholder*.

The clearest evidence that mental imagery is a trainable skill comes from sport psychology. Here it has been widely recognised that athletes are able to improve their ability to produce imagery with practice, and there are detailed guidelines in existence on how to hone one's visualisation skills.[89] Imagery training courses usually involve a stepwise approach, starting with simple tasks such as asking the participants to envisage how many windows their bedroom has and then gradually adding details to the picture (e.g. intricate features of the furniture), practising control (e.g. choosing the perspective or managing movement in the image) and adding other senses to visualisation (e.g. noises or typical smells). As a result, highly trained skiers, for example, are able to not only follow the complete course down the slope in their mind's eye, but can even make imagined "forced mistakes" which they can then correct, thereby practising trouble-shooting without actually endangering themselves.[90] Such mental rehearsal also works in fields other than sports; Kosslyn and Moulton, for example, describe how a medical team prepared for a complex operation to separate conjoined twins who were born joined at the tops of their heads, and cite one of the doctors:

> I do the case in my head, I must have done it 100 times. Every time, a problem would come up and I would find a solution and do it again. Every time I ran it in my head, it went faster. I'm sure everybody did the case 100 times.[91]

Finally, Robertson recounts reports that the world-renowned concert pianist Glenn Gould did very little actual piano practise in the last stages of his career, but he read the score and mentally rehearsed it several times instead. He would even make recordings of music that he had practised only in his mind.[92]

Enhancing the motivational power of vision

There have been several well-documented attempts in educational psychology to design vision-enhancing programmes with the specific aim of

89 For an authoritative summary published by the American Psychological Association, see Gould et al., "Imagery Training."
90 E.g. Weinberg and Gould (*Sport and Exercise Psychology*, 311) cite Sylvie Bernier, an Olympic champion in springboard diving: "It took me a long time to control my images and perfect my imagery, maybe a year, doing it every day. At first I couldn't see myself; I always saw everyone else, or I would see my dives wrong all the time. I would get an image of hurting myself, or tripping on the board, or I would see something done really bad. As I continued to work on it, I got to the point where I could see myself doing a perfect dive and the crowd at the Olympics. But it took me a long time."
91 Kosslyn and Moulton, "Mental Imagery and Implicit Memory," 37.
92 Robertson, *The Mind's Eye*, 205.

increasing the commitment of undermotivated student cohorts, such as inner city minority students in the US. One recurring finding has been that although vision does have the capacity to motivate action in various school contexts, this does not always happen automatically but depends on a number of conditions.[93] For the purpose of the current book, six of the lessons drawn from these educational interventions are particularly relevant:

- The vision needs to *exist*. The primary and obvious prerequisite for the motivational capacity of a vision is that it is available for people to pursue. The absence of sufficient motivation in many people is simply due to the fact that they do not have a sufficiently developed vision.
- The vision needs to be *elaborate* and *vivid*. The more intricate and detailed a future image, the more likely it will become an effective motivator, and the reverse is also true: images with insufficient specificity and detail will fail to evoke a strong enough motivational response.
- The vision needs to be perceived as *plausible*. The envisaged future scenario must be both realistic and perceived to be within the individual's competence. Plausibility is an essential prerequisite for motivation since implausible images are likely to remain at the level of unregulated fantasy without any motivational force.
- The vision needs to be regularly *activated* in the individual's mind. Even when a future image is both vivid and plausible, it only becomes relevant for behaviour when it is repeatedly primed in one's mind by various reminders, so that the vision does not get side-lined by other life concerns.
- The vision needs to be accompanied by a blueprint of concrete *pathways* (i.e. strategies, subgoals and action plans) that will lead to the desired future state. The availability of such a roadmap makes the difference between a motivationally relevant vision and an empty daydream or fantasy.
- The vision exerts maximum motivational impact if people also have a vivid image of the *negative consequences* of failing to achieve the desired endstate. The "pushing power" of these feared images will effectively complement the pulling power of the desired vision.

Having identified the relevant prerequisites to the motivational capacity of vision, an obvious way of enhancing imagery skills is to make sure that these conditions are met. In our book on building vision with a special focus on language classrooms, Maggie Kubanyiova and I proposed a six-phase vision-enhancing training approach,[94] assigning a macrostrategy to each

---

93 For a review, see Dörnyei and Ushioda, *Teaching and Researching Motivation*, 83–84.
94 Dörnyei and Kubanyiova, *Motivating Learners*, 32.

main motivational condition and then breaking these down to further specific techniques:

- The learner has a vision. → *Creating the vision*. People can be helped to develop a vision by participating in regular taster sessions of what the desired future state will be like. These may involve real experiences or mental simulations through guided imagery, guided narratives (to achieve a transformation experience) or observing influential role models.
- The vision is elaborate and vivid. → *Strengthening the vision through imagery enhancement*. In order to strengthen the vision, people can participate in various forms of visualisation skills training, either in an organised manner or as a personal exercise. In educational contexts, the power of virtual worlds can also be harnessed (e.g. through computer programs involving avatars). Another effective way of strengthening the learners' individual vision is to generate and enhance the collective vision of the whole group they belong to.
- The vision is perceived as plausible. → *Substantiating the vision by making it plausible*. We can make the vision plausible by anchoring it in reality, through encouraging honest reality self-checks, cultivating realistic beliefs (rather than illusions) and confronting – and then hopefully eliminating – any possible obstacles and barriers. In this way we can avoid the inherent danger associated with vision formation, namely the construction of a "story of self-deception," made up of projections of unrealistic desires.
- The vision is accompanied by effective procedural strategies. → *Transforming the vision into action*. In order to achieve this, people can map out pathways to success through visualisation (i.e. process imagery) and can then receive individual guidance on their action plans from an advisor.
- The vision is regularly activated. → *Keeping the vision alive*. The vision can be primed through regular reminders and prompts that are related to the desired goal, and by re-envisaging any outdated or "out-of-sync" images.
- The learner is also aware of the negative consequences of not achieving the vision. → *Counterbalancing the vision by considering failure*. This can involve regular reminders of the negative consequences of not succeeding as well as integrating images of feared possible selves into visualisation tasks. This practice, however, raises an important ethical dilemma: while visualising personal failure is undoubtedly a robust "scare tactic," one may argue that its negative effects on the self-esteem of some people can be so damaging that it takes the "counterbalancing" act too far. Let us consider this issue in a bit more detail.

How much to "rock the boat"

It is an age-old question whether an intervention should rely solely or primarily on the pulling power of a positive incentive (i.e. the "carrot") or the pushing power of a negative consequence that someone wants to avoid (i.e. the "stick"). A Christian analogy would be the evangelistic dilemma as to whether one should only highlight the prospect of spending eternity in the Father's house or also the alternative of the "fire and brimstone" of hell. Motivational psychology has recognized this contrast by distinguishing between *approach* versus *avoidance* motivation,[95] and the psychological considerations about which of the two engenders more intensive human transformation go somewhat against the contemporary "focus-on-the-positive" zeitgeist: as will be illustrated, profound conceptual change often requires some degree of initial "rocking the boat." Adapted from Maggie Kubanyiova's theory of conceptual change in teacher cognition,[96] the following extended metaphorical image summarises the main principles in this respect:[97]

Inspired by the title of John Ortberg's book *If You Want to Walk on Water, You Need to Get Out of the Boat*,[98] let us imagine a training course focusing on "Walking on Water." The participants are sitting in their small boats in the middle of a lake, intently listening to what the instructor has to say. There is a lot of excitement and fervent engagement with the topic as they are made familiar with the latest developments in the art of walking on water. But when the invitation finally comes from the trainer to come and try walking on water for themselves, many (if not most) choose to remain in their boats. The question is, why? Some are just having a nice outdoor experience on the lake, and although they are really enjoying the course, they never really thought of themselves as water-walkers and, to be honest, never really intended to learn, let alone use, this skill in their lives. Some others are convinced that they have already mastered the technique and, therefore, while in total agreement with what the trainer has to say, are certain that the invitation is not really for them but for their novice peers. Finally, a small group of trainees may begin to respond to the call and may even find the courage to try to step out of the boat, but as soon as their feet touch the water, they realise how cold, deep and dangerous the water really is, and thus quickly return to the safety of their boats. So, the question is, how can the trainees be better equipped to get out of their boats? In order to bring about conceptual change, there are three crucial intervention components to consider:

(a) *Inspire a vision (resonance).* The course participants are unlikely to feel the need to get out of the boat if the course content does not *resonate*

95 See e.g. Elliot, "Approach and Avoidance Motivation," 3.
96 Kubanyiova, *Teachers' Conceptual Change.*
97 Dörnyei and Kubanyiova, *Motivating Learners,* 27–28.
98 Ortberg, *If You Want to Walk on Water.*

with their vision of who they want to become. They need to see themselves as potential water-walkers.

(b) *Rock the boat (dissonance).* People can hardly live up to their visions by staying put, but the perceived risk of drowning can be debilitating. Only a certain amount of dissonance will dislodge them, and therefore the course leader must (gently) rock the boat and (slowly) shake the participants out of their comfort zones.

(c) *Spread a safety net (hope).* Rocking the boat when all the course participants can see is rough and dangerous waters can be a genuinely frightening experience. However, spreading safety nets and providing plenty of models and practice runs can turn the threat into a challenge and give the participants *hope* that walking on water is not something people are born with, but rather a skill that anyone can develop if they learn to trust their vision and persevere in their practice.

Summary

This chapter began with a description of the fluctuation in scientific respectability that the study of mental imagery has been subject to. After an initial heyday during the genesis of modern psychology at the turn of the 20th century, it fell out of favour during the behaviourist period, although maintaining its significance in clinical psychology because of its capacity to uncover aspects of the unconscious mind. The subject was reclaimed by academic psychology only from the 1960s onwards as a result of converging interests in brain research, psychopharmacology (due to the spread of psychedelic drugs) and cognitive psychology (because of its links to various memory functions). Currently the study of mental simulation and rehearsal enjoys high academic prestige in a number of areas within the social sciences, from psychology to business studies, with its applications utilised in fields as diverse as sport, education and psychotherapy.

The field of business management has adopted an extended notion of vision, referring to an ideal image of a future state that has strong motivational connotations. That is, vision in the world of business is almost always associated with aspirations to greatness, and the potency of any specific vision is seen to be reflected in the degree to which people embrace it. This emphasis foregrounded the shared, collective aspect of vision and the medium through which it is communicated, the vision statement. It was found that an effective vision statement needs to: offer a vivid description of a better place; convey enthusiasm and excitement; be inclusive in nature so that participants can find their own dreams in it; reflect the organisation's core ideology; and offer a clear finish line to shoot for.

The motivational dimension of vision is not, however, restricted to the field of business and leadership studies. It was argued that the act of conjuring up mental pictures, particularly scenes of imagined future realities, can be used to inspire and energise people more generally across a broad spectrum of life activities. Indeed, psychological research has identified several channels through which the human faculty to imagine future events can positively impact human behaviour, for example linking it to ideal self-images and arousing positive emotions. While there is almost complete agreement that vision can generate motivation, scholarly opinions differ about how and to what extent the image of a successful outcome can also provide directions to channel the generated energy into constructive goal-related behaviour.

Nevertheless, research on vision in the social sciences has been wide-ranging, producing a wealth of findings and transferrable lessons. Of these, the strategies established in sport, psychotherapy and educational psychology are particularly relevant for the current book. While the concluding section of this chapter has provided an overview of how these strategies can enhance visionary skills and the motivational power of vision, this topic will also be revisited in more practical detail in the final two chapters of the book.

References

Arbuthnott, Katherine D., Dennis W. Arbuthnott, and Lucille Rossiter. 2001. "Guided Imagery and Memory: Implications for Psychotherapists." *Journal of Counseling Psychology* 48, no. 2: 123–32.

Baddeley, Alan D., and Jackie Andrade. 2000. "Working Memory and the Vividness of Imagery." *Journal of Experimental Psychology: General* 129, no. 1: 126–45.

Baumeister, Roy F., Kathleen D. Vohs, C. Nathan DeWall, and Liqing Zhang. 2007. "How Emotion Shapes Behavior: Feedback, Anticipation, and Reflection, Rather Than Direct Causation." *Personality and Social Psychology Review* 11, no. 2: 167–203.

Berg, Jodi L. 2015. "The Role of Personal Purpose and Personal Goals in Symbiotic Visions." *Frontiers in Psychology* 6, no. 443: 1–13.

Boyatzis, Richard E., and Kleio Akrivou. 2006. "The Ideal Self as the Driver of Intentional Change." *Journal of Management Development* 25, no. 7: 624–42.

Clark, Brian C., Niladri K. Mahato, Masato Nakazawa, Timothy D. Law, and James S. Thomas. 2014. "The Power of the Mind: The Cortex as a Critical Determinant of Muscle Strength/Weakness." *Journal of Neurophysiology* 112: 3219–26.

Collins, James C., and Jerry I. Porras. 1996. "Building Your Company's Vision." *Harvard Business Review* 74, no. 5: 65–77.

Cox, Richard H. 2012. *Sport Psychology: Concepts and Applications*. 7th ed. New York: McGraw-Hill.

Crites, Stephen. "The Narrative Quality of Experience." *Journal of the American Academy of Religion* 39, no. 3 (1971): 291–311.

Curtis, Rebecca. 2016. "The Use of Imagery in Psychoanalysis and Psychotherapy." *Psychoanalytic Inquiry* 36, no. 8: 593–602.

Dörnyei, Zoltán. 2014. "Future Self-Guides and Vision." In *The Impact of Self-Concept on Language Learning*, edited by K. Csizér and M. Magid, 7–18. Bristol: Multilingual Matters.

Dörnyei, Zoltán. 2018. *Progressive Creation and Humanity's Struggles in the Bible: A Canonical Narrative Interpretation*. Eugene, OR: Pickwick.

Dörnyei, Zoltán, Alastair Henry, and Christine Muir 2016. *Motivational Currents in Language Learning: Frameworks for Focused Interventions*. New York: Routledge.

Dörnyei, Zoltán, and Maggie Kubanyiova. 2014. *Motivating Learners, Motivating Teachers: Building Vision in the Language Classroom*. Cambridge: Cambridge University Press.

Dörnyei, Zoltán, and Ema Ushioda. 2011. *Teaching and Researching Motivation.* 2nd ed. Harlow: Longman.

Dunkel, Curtis, and Jennifer Kerpelman, eds. 2006. *Possible Selves: Theory, Research, and Applications.* New York: Nova Science.

Elliot, Andrew J. 2008. "Approach and Avoidance Motivation and Achievement Goals." In *Handbook of Approach and Avoidance Motivation*, edited by A. J. Elliot, 3–14. New York: Psychology Press.

Epstein, Seymour. 1998. *Constructive Thinking: The Key to Emotional Intelligence.* Westport, CT: Greenwood.

Epstude, Kai, and Neal J. Roese. 2008. "The Functional Theory of Counterfactual Thinking." *Personality and Social Psychology Review* 12, no. 2: 168–92.

Feltz, Deborah L., and Daniel M. Landers. 1983. "The Effects of Mental Practice on Motor Skill Learning and Performance: A Meta-Analysis." *Journal of Sport Psychology* 5: 25–57.

Galton, Francis. 1880. "Statistics of Mental Imagery." *Mind: A Quarterly Review of Psychology and Philosophy* 19, no. 8: 301–18.

Galton, Francis. 1892/1907. *Inquiries into Human Faculty and Its Development.* 2nd ed. London: J. M. Dent & Co.

Gould, Daniel, Nicole Damarjian, and Christy Greenleaf. 2002. "Imagery Training for Peak Performance." In *Exploring Sport and Exercise Psychology*, edited by J. L. Van Raalte and B. W. Brewer, 49–74. Washington, DC: American Psychological Association.

Green, Melanie C., and Timothy C. Brock. 2000. "The Role of Transportation in the Persuasiveness of Public Narratives." *Journal of Personality and Social Psychology* 79, no. 5: 701–21.

Green, Melanie C., and John K. Donahue. 2009. "Simulated Worlds: Transportation into Narratives.". In *Handbook of Imagination and Mental Stimulation*, edited by K. Markman, W. M. P. Klein and J. A. Suhr, 241–54. New York: Psychology Press.

Gregg, Melanie, and Craig Hall. 2006. "Measurement of Motivational Imagery Abilities in Sport." *Journal of Sports Sciences* 24, no. 9: 961–71.

Hall, Craig R., Diane E. Mack, Allan Paivio, and Heather A. Hausenblas. 1998. "Imagery Use by Athletes: Development of the Sport Imagery Questionnaire." *International Journal of Sport Psychology* 29: 73–89.

Hall, Eric, Carol Hall, Pamela Stradling, and Diane Young. 2006. *Guided Imagery: Creative Interventions in Counselling and Psychotherapy.* London: Sage.

Higgins, E. Tory. 1987. "Self-Discrepancy: A Theory Relating Self and Affect." *Psychological Review* 94: 319–40.

Holmes, Emily A., and Andrew Matthews. 2010. "Mental Imagery in Emotion and Emotional Disorders." *Clinical Psychology Review* 30: 349–62.

Holt, Robert R. 1964. "Imagery: The Return of the Ostracized." *American Psychologist* 19, no. 4: 254–64.

Hoyle, Rick H., and Michelle R. Sherrill. 2006. "Future Orientation in the Self-System: Possible Selves, Self-Regulation, and Behavior." *Journal of Personality* 74, no. 6: 1673–96.

Ji, Julie L., Stephanie Burnett Heyes, Colin MacLeod, and Emily A. Holmes. 2016. "Emotional Mental Imagery as Simulation of Reality: Fear and Beyond – a Tribute to Peter Lang." *Behavior Therapy* 47: 702–19.

Kosslyn, Stephen M., and Samuel T. Moulton. 2009. "Mental Imagery and Implicit Memory." In *The Handbook of Imagination and Mental Simulation*, edited by K. Markman, W. M. P. Klein and J. A. Suhr, 35–51. New York: Psychology Press.

Kouzes, James M., and Barry Z. Posner. 2017. *The Leadership Challenge: How to Make Extraordinary Things Happen in Organisations.* 6th ed. Hoboken, NJ: Wiley.

Kubanyiova, Maggie. 2012. *Teacher Development in Action: Understanding Language Teachers' Conceptual Change.* Basingstoke, UK: Palgrave Macmillan.

Kurland, Hanna, Hilla Peretz, and Rachel Hertz-Lazarowitz. 2010. "Leadership Style and Organizational Learning: The Mediate Effect of School Vision." *Journal of Educational Administration* 48, no. 1: 7–30.

Lebon, Florent, Christian Collet, and Aymeric Guillot. 2010. "Benefits of Motor Imagery Training on Muscle Strength." *Journal of Strength and Conditioning Research* 24, no. 6: 1680–87.

Leondari, Angeliki, Efi Syngollitou, and Grigoris Kiosseoglou. 1998. "Academic Achievement, Motivation and Future Selves." *Educational Studies* 24, no. 2: 153–63.

Levin, Ira M. 2000. "Vision Revisited: Telling the Story of the Future." *Journal of Applied Behavioral Science* 36, no. 1: 91–107.

Markus, Hazel, and Paula Nurius. 1986. "Possible Selves." *American Psychologist* 41: 954–69.

Markus, Hazel, and Paula Nurius. 1987. "Possible Selves: The Interface between Motivation and the Self-Concept". In *Self and Identity: Psychosocial Perspectives* edited by K. Yardley and T. Honess, 157–72. Chichester: John Wiley & Sons.

Markus, Hazel, and Ann Ruvolo. 1989. "Possible Selves: Personalized Representations of Goals." In *Goal Concepts in Personality and Social Psychology*, edited by L. A. Pervin, 211–41. Hillsdale, NJ: Lawrence Erlbaum.

Maslow, Abraham H. 1968. *Toward a Psychology of Being.* 2nd ed. New York: D. Van Nostrand.

McMahon, C. E. 1973. "Images as Motives and Motivators: A Historical Perspective." *American Journal of Psychology* 86, no. 3: 465–90.

Meugnot, Aurore, and Nounagnon Frutueux Agbangla. 2015. "Motor Imagery Practice May Compensate for the Slowdown of Sensorimotor Processes Induced by Short-Term Upper-Limb Immobilization." *Psychological Research* 79: 489–99.

Morris, Tony. 2010. "Imagery." In *Routledge Handbook of Applied Sport Psychology: A Comprehensive Guide for Students and Practitioners* edited by Stephanie J. Hanrahan and Mark B. Andersen, 481–89. Abingdon: Routledge.

Munroe-Chandler, Krista J., and Michelle D. Guerrero. 2017. "Psychological Imagery in Sport and Performance." In *Oxford Research Encyclopedia of Psychology (Online)*, edited by Oliver Braddick. Oxford: Oxford University Press.

Ortberg, John. 2001. *If You Want to Walk on Water, You've Got to Get out of the Boat.* Grand Rapids, MI: Zondervan.

Oyserman, Daphna, and Leah James. 2009. "Possible Selves: From Content to Process." In *The Handbook of Imagination and Mental Simulation*, edited by K. Markman, W. M. P. Klein and J. A. Suhr, 373–94. New York: Psychology Press.

Pillemer, David. 2003. "Directive Functions of Autobiographical Memory: The Guiding Power of the Specific Episode." *Memory* 11, no. 2: 193–202.

Ranganathan, Vinoth K., Vlodek Siemionow, Jing Z. Liu, Vinod Sahgal, and Guang H. Yue. 2004. "From Mental Power to Muscle Power – Gaining Strength by Using the Mind." *Neuropsychologia* 42: 944–56.

Reeve, Johnmarshall. 2015. *Understanding Motivation and Emotion.* 6th ed. Hoboken, NJ: Wiley.

Reiser, Mathias, Dirk Büsch, and Jörn Munzert. 2011. "Strength Gains by Motor Imagery with Different Ratios to Physical to Mental Practice." *Frontiers in Psychology* 2, no. 194: 1–8.

Robertson, Ian. 2002. *The Mind's Eye: An Essential Guide to Boosting Your Mental Power*. London: Bantam Books.

Rogers, Carl R. 1965. *Client-Centered Therapy: Its Current Practice, Implications, and Theory*. Boston, MA: Houghton Mifflin.

Samuels, Mike, and Nancy Samuels. 1975. *Seeing with the Mind's Eye: The History, Techniques and Uses of Visualization*. New York: Random House.

Singer, Jerome L. 2006. *Imagery in Psychotherapy*. Washington, DC: American Psychological Association.

Slimani, Maamer, David Tod, Helmi Chaabene, Bianca Miarka, and Karim Chamari. 2016. "Effects of Mental Imagery on Muscular Strength in Healthy and Patient Participants: A Systematic Review." *Journal of Sports Science and Medicine* 15: 434–50.

Stam, Daan, Daan van Knippenberg, and Barbara Wisse. 2010. "Focusing on Followers: The Role of Regulatory Focus and Possible Selves in Visionary Leadership." *Leadership Quarterly* 21: 457–68.

Strange, Jill M., and Michael D. Mumford. 2002. "The Origins of Vision: Charismatic Versus Ideological Leadership." *Leadership Quarterly* 13: 343–77.

Taylor, Shelley E., Lien B. Pham, Inna D. Rivkin, and David A. Armor. 1998. "Harnessing the Imagination: Mental Simulation, Self-Regulation, and Coping." *American Psychologist* 53, no. 4: 429–39.

Thomas, Valerie. 2016. *Using Mental Imaging in Counselling and Psychotherapy: A Guide to More Inclusive Theory and Practice*. Abingdon: Routledge.

Tomkins, Silvan S. 2008. *Affect, Imagery, Consciousness: The Complete Edition*. New York: Springer.

van der Helm, R. 2009. "The Vision Phenomenon: Towards a Theoretical Underpinning of Visions of the Future and the Process of Envisioning." *Futures* 41: 96–104.

Vasquez, Noelia A., and Roger Buehler. 2007. "Seeing Future Success: Does Imagery Perspective Influence Achievement Motivation?" *Personality and Social Psychology Bulletin* 33: 1392–405.

Weinberg, Robert S., and Daniel Gould. 2015. *Foundations of Sport and Exercise Psychology*. 6th ed. Champaign, IL: Human Kinetics.

Yao, Wan X., Vinoth K. Ranganathan, Didier Allexandre, Vlodek Siemionow, and Guang H. Yue. 2013. "Kinesthetic Imagery Training of Forceful Muscle Contractions Increases Brain Signal and Muscle Strength." *Frontiers in Human Neuroscience* 7, no. 561: 1–6.

3 Vision in Scripture

The previous two chapters have demonstrated that vision is a high-profile concept in various psychological research domains, and that the potency of vision has been explored in fields as diverse as psychotherapy, business management, education and sports. As we turn now to examining the theological aspects of the notion, we shall see that vision is also an important *biblical* concept that occurs frequently in the Scriptures, and which is involved in some of the key episodes of the biblical narrative. In a similar way to how the notion of mental imagery was broadened in the scientific domain to include different modalities and cognitive functions, visionary experiences in the Bible also subsume a much wider scope than one would initially expect: not only did Old Testament prophets such as Ezekiel, Zechariah and Daniel perceive vivid images that originated from God – which would qualify as "visions" in the strictest sense – but the Bible also attributes the *hearing* of the word of the Lord to visionary experiences, as attested to, for example, by Genesis 15:1, where we read that "the word of the Lord came to Abram *in a vision*" (emphasis added; see also Psalm 89:19 for a similar construction). Indeed, in Numbers 12:6 God declares, "When there are prophets among you, I the Lord make myself known to them *in visions*" (emphasis added). This "visionary-hearing" experience is not restricted to the Old Testament, as in Acts 9:10 we read that the Lord spoke "in a vision" to Ananias and in Acts 18:9 also to Paul.

To further illustrate the potential richness of the biblical concept of vision, we should note that in the last example, Paul's vision took place at night ("One night the Lord said to Paul in a vision"), which raises the question as to whether this communication was part of a dream. If we look further, we find several examples in Scripture of the phrase "vision of the night" (e.g. Gen 46:2; Job 33:15), with Isaiah 29:7 specifically linking these to dreams: "like a dream, a vision of the night." In fact, the fluidity of the boundaries of the semantic domain of vision does not end here; vision-like experiences are also implied by other related terms such as "revelation" (e.g. in 2 Cor 12:1: "I will go on to visions and revelations of the Lord") or "trance" (e.g. in Acts 10:10–11 when Peter went up on the roof to pray, "he fell into a trance. He saw the heaven opened . . ."), and even angelic visitations (e.g. the encounter of John the Baptist's father, Zechariah, with an angel in the Temple is described in Luke 1:22 as a "vision" and when Peter was miraculously freed by an angel from prison, "he thought he was seeing a vision"; Acts 12:9).

It has also been noted by scholars that many visionary experiences described in the Bible are not marked by explicit "vision" terminology at all;[1] while some of these (e.g. Ezekiel's vision of the valley of the dry bones; 37:1–14) are straightforward visionary images in the strictest sense, commentators often identify other extended divine inspirations as "visions" proper, even when the text does not refer to any actual imagery experience. Perhaps the best example of this is the Book of Revelation as a whole, where the apocalyptic vision presented is only once referred to as a "vision" (in Rev 9:17).[2] Finally, in several places within the biblical corpus we come across usages of "seeing" and the phrase "opening someone's eyes" that appear to go beyond any form of literal, physical perception, pointing to the involvement of inner senses, not unlike those observed in cognitive neuroscience. Thus, while visionary experiences of various kinds are frequent in the Bible, it may not be entirely straightforward to decide what their exact make-up is or how they are related to each other. This is where the neuroscientific principles presented in the previous chapters can help to identify and categorise the different types; for example, we have seen that the same neural processes underlie the different modalities of mental imagery (such as inner seeing and inner hearing) or that the vision element in waking dreams and night-time dreams is similar. Psychological considerations will also be instrumental to extending the notion of biblical vision into new areas; to give here but one example, we shall see that God's description of the Promised Land meets the criteria of functioning as guided imagery proper.

In sum, the Scriptures are laced with descriptions of visionary experiences in both Testaments, and these experiences show considerable variation in terms of their exact nature and function. Therefore, the first task in exploring the notion of biblical vision is to take stock of the various vision-like occurrences in order to establish the scope of the phenomenon. After this survey, we shall address the important question of whether biblical prophets can be understood to operate in a "visionary mode" in general, and then explore what some biblical usages of "seeing" and "opening one's eyes" signify when they do not appear to be related to bodily perception. The chapter concludes with a discussion of how biblical vision reports may act as guided imagery by evoking visionary experiences in the audience.

1 See e.g. Stead, "Visions," 819; Miller, "Dreams and Visions," 217.
2 E.g. Everts, "Dreams," 231; however, as Aune ("Vision," 994) points out, the absence of "vision" terminology in Revelation is compensated by the frequent use of the phrase "I saw" (almost 40 times).

Various forms of vision in the Bible

The most straightforward aspect of biblical vision concerns examples when the term "vision" is explicitly mentioned in the Scriptures. However, as stated earlier, we also find related terms with overlapping semantic domains – most notably "dream," "revelation" and "trance" – signifying vision-like experiences, and in some instances the text presents what appear to be vision reports without using any specific vision terminology. Let us consider each of these categories separately.

Visions and auditions

The NRSV translation of the Bible contains over 100 occurrences of the word "vision(s)," and virtually all of these refer to some form of mental imagery, that is, "a psychological or revelatory experience in which the subject privately 'sees' that which is not physically present to ordinary unaided sense perception"[3] (Aune). All the Hebrew, Aramaic and Greek terms used in the original texts for authentic visions (i.e. not for false visions) have to do with words referring to "seeing" in contexts of normal visual perception,[4] and therefore they are in accordance with the way "vision" has been used in non-biblical contexts (as discussed earlier). These are thus unambiguous cases, and the second part of this chapter as well as Chapter 4 will provide an analysis of their meaning and functions.

David Aune further explains that although the various Hebrew and Aramaic terms for "vision" are primarily related to seeing in the biblical usage, *auditions* (i.e. auditory experiences) are also assumed under the term,[5] similar to how mental imagery subsumes both the visual and auditory modalities. Indeed, starting with Genesis we find that "the word of the Lord came to Abram in a vision" (15:1) and "God spoke to Israel in a vision at night" (46:2), and in a similar vein, the Lord's word is reported to have come "in a vision" to several prophets (e.g. Amos 1:1; Obad 1:1; Nah 1:1). Likewise, God's communication with King David is reported as "Then you spoke in a vision to your faithful one" (Psalm 89:19), and the young Samuel's hearing from the Lord for the first time is also described as a "vision" (1 Sam 3:15) even though no visual element is reported. In some places in the Old Testament, prophetic "words" and "vision" are used synonymously (e.g. 1 Sam 3:1; 1 Chr 17:15), and the reference to auditory stimuli through visual terminology is also present in the New Testament, for example when the Lord speaks both to Ananias and Paul "in a vision" (Acts 9:10 and 18:9) or,

---

3 Aune, "Vision," 993.
4 In Hebrew and Aramaic, cognates of *ḥzh* ("see"): *ḥāzôn, ḥāzôṯ, ḥāzûṯ, ḥizzāyô, maḥazeh, ḥŭzû* (Aramaic); and cognates of *rʾh* ("see"): *marʾâ, marʾeh, rōʾeh*. In Greek: *hórama* and *hórasis* (from *horáō*, "to see") and *optasía* (from *optánomai*, "look at"); see ibid., 993–994.
5 Ibid., 994.

as Edith Humphrey underlines, in the curious phraseology of Acts 22:18, where Paul recounts that he "saw Jesus saying to me. . . ."[6] Thus, Hanson rightly concludes that "not only did no specific terminology for auditions develop, but that even where the dream-vision proper is only auditory, visual terminology prevails."[7]

Dreams

The Hebrew word for "dream" (*chlwm*) and its Aramaic cognate (*chlm* in Dan 2–5) are used in the Old Testament to refer to both ordinary dreams and oracular dreams (i.e. message dreams with vision content). In the New Testament two different Greek words appear (*onar* and *enypnion*) which could have both oracular or non-oracular meanings in classical Greek, even though in the Scriptures they are used only in the former, oracular sense.[8] The question, then, is whether the visionary content of the oracular dreams is to be distinguished from visions as discussed earlier. Vision and dream have overlapping semantic domains in several modern languages (e.g. the English phrase used by Martin Luther King Jr., "I have a dream . . .," has nothing to do with sleep), and this intersecting usage also appears to be typical of the Scriptures: as mentioned earlier, sometimes the two words are used synonymously (e.g. Num 12:6; Job 7:14), and we also find several examples of the phrase "vision(s) of the night" (e.g. Gen 46:2; Dan 2:19), sometimes in a synonymous position with dream (e.g. Isa 29:7; Job 20:8; 33:15).

In other places, dream and vision are interchangeable: for example, in Daniel 7 we are told that Daniel had "a dream and visions of his head as he lay in bed" (v. 1), and he wrote down the "dream" (v. 1), which is then referred to as "vision by night" (v. 2, a term he repeats in v. 7), "night vision" (v. 13) and "vision of my head" (v. 15). Earlier, in Daniel 2:28, "dream" and "visions of the head" are also used as synonyms, and in Daniel 4:5 a further synonym, "fantasy," is added: "I saw a dream that frightened me; my fantasies in bed and the visions of my head terrified me." These examples should suffice to explain why there is a general consensus amongst scholars that waking visions, night visions and dream-visions are merely different forms of receiving similar types of revelatory content.[9] This is consistent with the neuroscientific characterisation of dreams as containing mental imagery of the same kind as daytime visualisations do (see Chapter 1).

The association between visions and dreams is further strengthened by the fact that "vision" and "night" are frequently linked together in the

---

6 Humphrey, *Rhetoric of Vision*, 85.
7 Hanson, "Dreams and Visions," 1411.
8 See e.g. Roberts, "Dream."
9 See e.g. Boyd, *Seeing Is Believing*, 85–86; Hanson, "Dreams and Visions," 1408; Miller, *Dreams and Visions in Luke-Acts*, 9; Miller, "Dreams and Visions," 216; Roberts, "Dream"; Stead, "Visions," 819.

Scriptures: prophets often receive visions at night (e.g. Isa 26:9; Zech 1:8), and Micah (3:6) describes the Lord's punishment of false prophets as "night will come over you, without visions" (NIV), implying that the default situation would be the opposite (i.e. night *with* vision). In the New Testament, Paul is reported to receive a vision at night – the message from the man of Macedonia (Acts 16:9) – which resulted in the gospel reaching Europe for the first time. Accordingly, Ryken, Wilhoit and Longman are right to conclude in the *Dictionary of Biblical Imagery* that "Night is the expected time to hear the voice of God or witness his revelation."[10] This is in accordance with the neuroscientific discussion of mental imagery earlier: because physical perception and mental imagery utilise the same region in the brain, the condition in which physical perception is less likely to cancel out internal imagery is either darkness or some state when conscious awareness is suspended, such as a dream.[11]

Revelations

We saw in the Introduction that vision and revelation are closely related notions (e.g. they are used as virtual synonyms in 2 Cor 12:1), because vision is a "revelatory medium" [12] (Aune). Interestingly, despite the theological significance of the concept of revelation, there is no specific technical term for it in Scripture. Instead, according to the *NIDNTTE*, we find in the New Testament a cluster of Greek words (and their cognates) that are frequently translated as "reveal" or "revelation,"[13] all used to refer to a variety of disclosure types, both in the ordinary and biblical/theological senses,[14] often pointing to the future in the passive (e.g. "when God's righteous judgment will be revealed"; Rom 2:5). In some cases they indicate concrete divine communication, either by specifying the medium of the message (e.g. it is revealed to the Magi in a dream-vision that they should not return to Herod; Matt 2:12) or without any specification (e.g. "It had been revealed to him [Simon] by the Holy Spirit that he would not die before he had seen the Lord's Messiah"; Luke 2:26).

In Galatians 1:12, Paul expresses very clearly the divine nature of his revelation ("I did not receive it [the gospel] from a human source, nor was I taught it, but I received it through a revelation of Jesus Christ"), and in other places he refers to this experience as a vision (e.g. Acts 26:19).

---

10 Ryken, Wilhoit and Longman, "Dreams, Visions," 217.
11 See e.g. Job 4:13: "Amid thoughts from visions of the night, when deep sleep falls on mortals."
12 Aune, "Vision," 994.
13 *Apokalypsis* (disclosure, revelation), *gnōrizō* (to make known), *dēloō* (to make clear, reveal), *epiphaneia* (appearance, revelation), *optanomai* (to be visible, appear), *horaō* (*pass.* appear, become visible), *phaneroō* (to reveal, show), *chrēmatizō* (to impart a revelation); see Silva, *NIDNTTE*, Vol.1, p. 69.
14 See Williams, "Revelation," 678.

Ephesians 1:17–18 provides an expressive illustration of the visionary element of revelation, likening the reception of revelation to the "enlightening of the eyes of one's heart." These examples underpin William Arnold's conclusion that we can understand visions "as instruments of supernatural revelation. They are audiovisual means of communication between a heavenly being and an earthly recipient."[15] Indeed, James Packer submits that "when the Bible speaks of revelation, the thought intended is of God the Creator actively disclosing to men his power and glory, his nature and character, his will, ways and plans."[16] We shall come back to this point when we discuss the functions of biblical vision in the next chapter.

In sum, the term "revelation" covers a broader semantic domain than that of "vision" used in this book, referring to, according to James Dunn, a spectrum from intellectual illumination through personal guidance to eschatological revelation.[17] Many of the revelatory experiences reported in the Scriptures can be directly or indirectly linked to perceptions of vision, but in most cases the focus of the text is on the outcome of revelation – that is, on the knowledge or information revealed – rather than on the process of how this happened.

Trances

When the Apostle Peter received the momentous vision of eating unclean animals on his rooftop, which eventually led to the acceptance of Gentiles amongst the followers of Christ, we are told that he "fell into a trance" (Acts 10:10). There are two further occurrences of the Greek word for trance (*ékstasis*) in the New Testament, with Acts 11:5 referring to the same event and Acts 22:17 describing Paul seeing a vision of Jesus talking to him in the Temple. Both occasions occurred during broad daylight, so in view of the neuroscientific considerations, it makes perfect sense that these examples of a "trance" – defined as a "mental state in which the person affected is partially or wholly unconscious of objective sensations, but intensely alive to subjective impressions"[18] (Macalister) – were to suspend Peter and Paul's conscious awareness in order to create cerebral space for the visionary experience. Allen Meyers, amongst others, also highlights 2 Corinthians 5:13 in this respect, where Paul states: "if we are beside ourselves,[19] it is for God; if we are in our right mind, it is for you." One interpretation of this verse is that Paul contrasts an altered state of consciousness – an ecstatic

---

15 Arnold, "Visions," 802–803.
16 Packer, "Revelation," 1014.
17 Dunn, "Biblical Concepts of Revelation," 14–15.
18 Macalister, "Trance," 3005.
19 According to the *NIDTTE*, the Greek word for being "beside oneself" (*existēmi*; "out of our mind"; NIV) is related to the noun *ékstasis*.

experience – that characterises some of his private relationship with God with his "right" (i.e. ordinary) mindset.[20]

With regard to the Old Testament, although there is no special Hebrew word used for trance, we come across a peculiar condition of "deep sleep" (*tardēmâ*) that is associated with visions in several places (Gen 15:12; Job 4:13; 33:15), referring to a state that is more profound than ordinary sleep[21] and which thus allows for uninterrupted vision experience. In some other places in Scripture, the verb "to prophesy" (*nābā'*) is connected with ecstatic behaviour (1 Sam 10:6, 10),[22] so much so that the NRSV, for example, translates it as being "in a prophetic frenzy."[23] Finally, the description of the prophet Balaam "falling down" is also likely to refer to a trance-like altered state of consciousness:

> the oracle of the man whose eye is clear,
> the oracle of one who hears the words of God,
> who sees the vision of the Almighty,
> who falls down, but with eyes uncovered
> (Num 24:3–4, repeated in 15–16)

In sum, there are a few occasions in the Scriptures where the perception of vision is accompanied by a trance-like state of altered consciousness. This is consistent with neuroscientific considerations, and in fact the curious aspect of these incidents is not so much why they occurred as why there are not many more examples of them in the biblical canon. We shall return to this issue later in a section that addresses religious experiences.

Visitations, apparitions and other heavenly irruptions into material reality

A unique category of the divine irrupting into human experience in the Bible involves the cases when people are visited by an angelic messenger. Do these instances take place on the visionary platform or do the angels become corporeal for the purpose of their visit and thus visible for bodily eyes?[24] This is a valid question, because we learn in Genesis 6:2 that the "sons of God" took human wives, which implies that spiritual beings are able to take material form. However, the Bible does not reveal any specific

---

20 E.g. Martin, *2 Corinthians*, 283–285; Thrall, *Second Corinthians*, 406.
21 The same state is mentioned in Gen 2:21 when God operated on Adam and created Eve of one of his ribs.
22 See Ashley, *Book of Numbers*, 213–214.
23 We shall see later that prophetic functions are closely linked to visionary experiences in general; because in these particular cases there is no explicit mention of an accompanying vision, we shall discuss them further under the rubric of "religious experience."
24 Groeschel (*Reported Revelations*, 156) calls such corporeal or ocular phenomena "exterior visions" on the basis that they can be experienced with bodily eyes.

details about the nature of these phenomena, and therefore we do not have a definite answer.[25] One possible way to clarify this issue further is to examine whether the angels are visual to everyone in their vicinity (in which case they may be considered "real") or only to the particular person involved (in which case they would be probably part of a private mental image). For example, during Paul's boat journey to Rome as a prisoner, the Apostle encouraged the sailors by telling them that "last night there stood by me an angel of the God . . ." (Acts 27:23–24), which was likely to be part of a personal vision or else others would have witnessed it in the relatively limited space of a boat. However, it is difficult to apply this test in most cases for several reasons:

(a) In some of the accounts virtually no information is given about the circumstances; for example, Acts 8:26 simply says, "Then an angel of the Lord said to Philip. . . ."
(b) Visitations often happen in private, without any onlookers; for example, when Zechariah (John the Baptist's father) was visited by the Archangel Gabriel, it happened in the innermost sanctuary of the Temple with no one else present (Luke 1:11–20) – in that case the text describes the event as a "vision" (v. 22).
(c) In some cases the onlookers can perceive partial or mixed reports of the phenomenon. For example, Matthew and Mark's accounts of Jesus' baptism report only Jesus seeing the Holy Spirit ascending on him as a dove (Matt 3:16 and Mark 1:10); in contrast, Luke (3:22) highlights the fact that "the Holy Spirit descended upon him *in bodily form* like a dove" (emphasis added), suggesting that it was visible to everybody, while John (1:32) only states that John the Baptist saw "the Spirit descending from heaven like a dove, and it remained on him." Regarding Paul's experience on the road to Damascus the picture is even less straightforward, because we have two contrasting accounts – "The men who were traveling with him stood speechless because they heard the voice but saw no one" (Acts 9:7) versus "Now those who were with me saw the light but did not hear the voice of the one who was speaking to me" (Acts 22:9) – suggesting that in the undoubtedly tumultuous situation Paul's companions were aware of some but not all of what he experienced.
(d) We do not know whether a mental vision can occur simultaneously to a group of people or only to a single individual. In Luke 24:4, several women are reported to have seen "two men in dazzling clothes" at Jesus

---

25 The ambiguity of this issue is illustrated by the fact that, as Groeschel (ibid., 157) points out, although most apparitions in church history appear to be mental imagery (or "imaginative vision" in his words), "the individual usually accepts them as part of the ordinary visual experience even though they contain unusual details. Often the visionaries report that the vision was extremely beautiful, unlike anything they have seen before."

tomb, which would suggest that this was a case of corporeal appearance, but the episode is later referred to as a "vision of angels" (v. 23). Similarly, the Transfiguration was witnessed by James, Peter and John and yet Jesus later described it as a "vision" (Matt 17:9).

Thus, we do not seem to have any firm basis to decide on the visionary nature of apparitions, and the best illustration of the dilemma between "real" and "unreal" in such cases is the Apostle Peter's miraculous freeing from prison by an angel, when "he did not realise that what was happening with the angel's help was real; he thought he was seeing a vision" (Acts 12:9). That is, Peter's default interpretation was that the apparition occurred at the mental rather than the physical level, whereas the text then suggests that he was wrong and "what was happening with the angel's help was real" (v. 9). In this respect, Leland Ryken and his colleagues conclude that "visions and angels coincided so often that the appearance of an angel suggests to Peter an 'unreal' state of mind."[26] In view of all these uncertainties, it is understandable that several scholars have chosen to include under the rubric of vision all "otherworldly encounters such as angelic appearances or a voice from heaven"[27] occurring in Scripture.

Vision-like scenes without any explicit vision terminology

Although many visitation scenes lack any specific vision terminology, they can still be considered to constitute a category of vision because the angelic presence in them serves as a clue that a heaven–earth encounter has taken place. There are, however, several other instances in the Bible which either appear to be vision reports or refer to outcomes of vision experiences without, offering any explicit textual clues that this was indeed the case. As an extreme, it was mentioned in the introduction of this chapter that even John's majestic vision described in the Book of Revelation is referred to as a "vision" only once (Rev 9:17). Another salient example concerns the making of the tabernacle: Exodus 26ff presents in great detail God's verbal instructions to Moses about what it should be like, but in Acts 7:44 Stephen suggests that Moses had the tabernacle prepared "according to the pattern he had *seen*" (emphasis added) – indeed, in Exodus we are told twice (25:9, 40) that God "showed" the "patterns" of the tabernacle to Moses.[28] Similarly, we read in 1 Chronicles 28 that King David handed

26 Ryken et al., "Dreams, Visions," 218.
27 Miller, "Dreams and Visions," 217; see also Aune, "Ecstasy," 15–16; Miller, *Dreams and Visions in Luke-Acts*, 10.
28 Brueggemann (*Theology of the Old testament*, 668) writes in this respect: "What strikes one repeatedly in this exposition of tabernacle, priesthood, mercy seat, and sacrificial system is the visual, material quality of everything that is authorized and proposed. . . . Moses and the workmen have available a model for their work. . . . The tabernacle and

over the detailed plans of the temple to Solomon, "the plan of all that he had in mind" (v. 12), with the same Hebrew word used for "plan" as for the tabernacle "patterns," and in v. 19 we also read, "All this, in writing at the Lord's direction, he made clear to me – the plan of all the works."[29] Thus, both Moses and David seem to have received an elaborate mental image and yet no vision vocabulary is employed in the text.

We also find several prophetic visions when an image is presented without being marked as a vision; for example, Stead highlights the fact that neither Ezekiel's vision of the valley of the dry bones (Ezek 37:1–14) nor Zechariah's night visions are described explicitly as "visions"[30] (although in the latter the context makes it clear that they are such), and neither is any vision terminology used in the New Testament when Stephen "gazed into heaven and saw the glory of God and Jesus standing at the right hand of God" (Acts 7:55). To cite a final cluster of examples, in several places in the Old Testament we are told about the word of the Lord coming to someone at night (to Nathan: 2 Sam 7:4 and 1 Chr 17:3; to Gideon: Judg 6:25 and 7:9; to Elijah: 1 Kgs 19:9), where we can assume the presence of a vision experience not only because of the earlier argument that auditions qualify as such but also because of the night context, which, as we have seen, constitutes the ideal condition for mental imagery in the absence of external visual distraction.

Prophetic vision

The Scriptures often report Old Testament prophets perceiving elaborate images that they could only have seen in their mind's eye. The most momentous of these images are the *theophanies*, that is, divine revelations in which God's presence is made visible and recognisable to humans; two pronounced examples are Isaiah 6:1–4 and Ezekiel 1:26–8, describing God sitting on his heavenly throne.[31] We also find many other visual images reported by prophets, some being symbolic or allegorical in the sense that they require interpretation (e.g. Amos 7:7–9; Dan 1–8; or Zechariah's multiple visions). There are however, some Old Testament prophets whose accounts do not contain any obvious imagery, with Jeremiah being the most prominent of these. As Pamela Scalise explains, although most interpreters would consider Jeremiah a visionary prophet, he reports very few actual images and does not authenticate his report with the technical language of visionary experience that we find in other prophetic accounts.[32] This raises the profound

all of the vehicles for presence are designed to appeal to the senses, and especially to visual sensibility."

29 Braun (*1 Chronicles*, 272) highlights the conscious allusion to the tabernacle narrative.
30 Stead, "Visions," 819.
31 According to Dunn ("Biblical Concepts of Revelation," 15), these served as "archetypes for subsequent mysticism."
32 Scalise, "Visions in Jeremiah," 47.

question as to whether there is an inherent link between being a prophet and functioning as a visionary.

1 Samuel 9:9 offers a rare linguistic insight into the origin of the word "prophet" when it is explained that "the one who is now called a prophet was formerly called a seer," and indeed, we find in the Old Testament almost two dozen references to prophets as "seers" (e.g. 1 Sam 9:19; 2 Sam 24:11; 1 Chr 25:5; 2 Chr 16:7; Amos 7:12). In other words, a traditional hallmark of prophets was that they could see "visions of the seer" (2 Chr 9:29). This is further confirmed by the fact that, as Benjamin Warfield, amongst others, has pointed out, the dominant verb of perception used in the Scriptures in relation to prophecy is not so much "to hear" as "to see":[33] Micah (1:1) "saw" the word of the Lord and so did Isaiah (2:1) and Amos (1:1). Isaiah (13:1) "saw" an oracle and so did Habakkuk (1:1). Habakkuk then further declared: "I will keep watch to see what he [the Lord] will say to me . . .," and when the Lord answered him, he was instructed to "Write the vision . . ." (2:2). In a similar vein, Jeremiah (38:20–22) declared, "Just obey the voice of the Lord in what I say to you . . . this is what the Lord has shown me – a vision . . .," and we also find a similar situation regarding Ezekiel (1:3): after "the word of the Lord came to the priest Ezekiel," the prophet started his account by saying, "As I looked . . ." (v. 4). Finally, when the young Samuel heard God's verbal message for the first time, the text simply refers to this as a "vision" (1 Sam 3:15).

Equally telling are in this respect some passages about false prophets: Ezekiel writes that they "follow their own spirit, and have seen nothing"; Jeremiah states that "They are prophesying to you a lying vision"; and in Lamentations 2:14 we read that "Your prophets have seen for you false and deceptive visions." Likewise, Isaiah declares about the prophets who are responsible for the blindness of the people: "he [the Lord] has closed your eyes, you prophets, and covered your heads, you seers. The vision of all this has become for you like the words of a sealed document" (29:10–11). Moreover, in 1 Samuel 3:1 we are told that "In those days the word of the Lord was rare; there were not many visions" (NIV), indicating that hearing the word of the Lord and visionary experiences were inextricably linked together. This is also expressed by the fact that in some places a prophet's overall prophecy is simply summarised as "vision"; for example, the entire book of Isaiah is labelled as "the vision . . . that Isaiah the prophet saw"[34] (Isa 1:1), and Hezekiah's story is concluded in 2 Chronicles 32:32 as follows: "The other events of Hezekiah's reign and his acts of devotion are written in the vision of the prophet Isaiah." Similarly, Nahum's prophecy begins with "The book of the vision of Nahum" (Nah 1:1) and the book of Obadiah with "The vision of Obadiah. This is what the Sovereign Lord says. . . ."

33 Warfield, "Revelation," 2578.
34 See Stead, "Visions," 818.

Thus, we have a curious situation that even though the Lord's action of communicating to the prophets is described in the Old Testament by the formula "Thus says the Lord" over 400 times, the perception of this message by humans appears to take place in a visionary mode, and the dominant verb to refer to the act of this perception is "see." This is, however, not a contradiction in the light of the previous two chapters, which have shown that auditions are a modality of mental imagery. We may therefore conclude that the prophetic "hearing" of the Lord's message may rightly be regarded as a visionary act, and this correspondence between prophecy and visionary perception is at the heart of Walter Brueggemann's general proposal about the "prophetic imagination." As he submits,

> the characteristic way of a prophet in Israel is that of poetry and lyric. The prophet engages in futuring fantasy. The prophet does not ask if the vision can be implemented, for questions of implementation are of no consequence until the vision can be imagined. . . . It is the vocation of the prophet to keep alive the ministry of imagination.[35]

We shall return to the prophetic function of creating an alternative world of possibilities in the next chapter, when we discuss the motivational function of divine vision.

"Seeing" and "opening one's eyes"

At the end of the Book of Job, God answers Job in two divine speeches, and consequently Job repents:

> I had heard of you by the hearing of the ear,
> but now my eye sees you;
> therefore I despise myself,
> and repent in dust and ashes.
> (Job 42:5–6)

The use of the verb "see" by Job in this important passage clearly refers to his internal vision rather than his physical sight, and the text declares that it is this deeper "seeing" which has led Job to a profound change of heart. Using "to see" with such a special meaning is not unique to this passage. When Simeon took the baby Jesus in his arms in the Temple, he proclaimed, "my eyes have seen your salvation, . . . a light for revelation to the Gentiles and for glory to your people Israel" (Luke 2:30–32), and Isaiah also speaks about "seeing" the salvation of the Lord (52:10; also cited in Luke 3:6) as well as "seeing" the glory of the Lord (40:5). These instances refer to

---

35 Brueggemann, *Prophetic Imagination*, 40.

beholding divine insights that only one's inner senses can perceive, a perception that is expressively referred to as the enlightenment of "the eyes of the heart" in a prayer at the beginning of Ephesians (1:17–19; emphasis added):

> I pray that the God of our Lord Jesus Christ, the Father of glory, may give you a spirit of wisdom and *revelation* as you come to know him, so that, with *the eyes of your heart enlightened*, you may know what is the hope to which he has called you, what are the riches of his glorious inheritance among the saints, and what is the immeasurable greatness of his power for us who believe, according to the working of his great power.

The significance of the enlightenment of the "eyes of the heart" is further evidenced in verses of Scripture that highlight the limitations or absence of the functioning of one's spiritual senses. Most notably, in 2 Corinthians 4:4 Paul emphasises the unbelievers' inability to see – "The god of this world has blinded the minds of unbelievers, to keep them from seeing the light of the gospel of the glory of Christ, who is the image of God" (2 Cor 4:4) – and Gregory Boyd captures the gist of the passage when he concludes that "the ability to see that believers have and unbelievers lack is *a seeing in the mind*"[36] (emphasis in the original).

The phrase "to open one's eyes" occurs frequently in the biblical corpus, sometimes referring to actual seeing,[37] sometimes to pleading to God to open his eyes to the prayers/plights of the petitioner,[38] but in several instances the text refers to an added dimension of seeing. For example, the Lord opened Hagar's eyes so that she could see the well (Gen 2:19); he also opened Balaam's eyes so that he could see an angel blocking the road (Numbers 22:31); and in 2 Kings 6:17 we are told that when Elisha prayed to the Lord to open the eyes of his servant, the latter was able to see God's army around them – it is particularly noteworthy in this last example that the prophet himself was obviously able to "see" this army even before that. The deeper meaning of the phrase is most explicit in Paul's commission by Jesus: in Acts 26:18 we read that Paul was sent to the Gentiles "to open their eyes so that they may turn from darkness to light." Here "seeing" may be equated with beholding the truth of Jesus, and the episode of the two disciples meeting Jesus on the road to Emmaus indicates that this interpretation may not be farfetched: although they did not initially recognise Jesus, after Jesus "interpreted to them the things about himself in all the scriptures" (Luke 24:27) and then "took bread, blessed and broke it, and gave it to them, . . . their eyes were opened, and they recognized him" (vv. 30–31;

36 Boyd, *Seeing Is Believing*, 88
37 E.g. in Matt 9:30, Jesus heals blind men by opening their eyes.
38 E.g. Neh 1:6.

ironically, as soon as they were able to see the true Jesus, "he vanished from their sight"; v. 31).

Vision reports and guided imagery in the Scriptures

When we talk about "biblical vision," the phrase can refer both to the visionary experiences of the recipients (usually prophets) and to the written accounts of these experiences recorded in the Scriptures. This twofold nature of vision (i.e. the actual experience and its report) has been summarised clearly by Ian Paul in his recent commentary on Revelation: "Did John have a vision (or series of visions)? If he did, he has reported it in a very careful way. We don't have a vision; we have a vision report, a text, and we should attend to it."[39] We saw in Chapter 2 that the overall quality of a vision in the business world depends not so much on the vividness of the original perception of the mental image as on the expressiveness of the vision statement. That is, the value of a business vision is measured by the degree to which it can impact people, and the same principle may apply to a biblical vision report, as indicated by how Ian Paul continues his argument:

> John's aim is not to impress us with his visionary experience, nor (necessarily) to encourage us to have our own. Rather, John wants us to order our lives in the light of the truth about God that these vision reports reveal to us.[40]

So far the focus in the current book has been largely on primary visionary experiences rather than how these are described by the recipients, but a survey of the biblical records of vision also necessitates the consideration of the nature of the written vision reports, because these cannot be regarded as equivalent to the original visions for several reasons:[41]

- *Private nature.* Vision is an inherently individual and private experience, and this inevitably adds a subjective element to any vision account that is hard to pin down because of the absence of any objective criteria.
- *Alternative reality.* The personal subjectivity in describing a vision is likely to be made more pronounced by the fact that divine vision concerns an alternative reality which is outside the receiver's familiar domain of operation; as Lyons puts it, the recipient experiences things "that are not normally experienced – sights of the deity and the heavenly realm, scenes of past or future events, encounters with heavenly

---

39 Paul, *Revelation*, 24.
40 Ibid., 24–25.
41 See e.g. Hayes and Tiemeyer, *Dream and Vision Reports in the Hebrew Bible*; Humphrey, *Rhetoric of Vision*; Proudfoot, *Religious Experience*; Rowland, "Visionary Experience."

beings, and travel to other (even cosmic) locations."[42] It is therefore not a straightforward task to decide how to make sense of these experiences and how best to convey their meaning to others.

- *Adaptation to a different medium.* A written vision report such as the biblical accounts of divine vision requires, by definition, the transformation of the original "audiovisual" imagery into verbal language.[43] The renowned German visionary, Hildegard of Bingen (1098–1179), described this duality in a letter as follows: "What I see and hear in the vision I write down. . . . The words I see and hear in the vision are not like the words that sound from a human mouth, but they are like shooting flame and a cloud moved in clear air."[44] Thus, the verbalisation process inevitably involves a degree of mediation and interpretation.[45]

- *Artistic creativity.* In order to do justice to the complex visionary experience that often involves multiple modalities, visionaries need to utilise the full repertoire of the linguistic and rhetorical devices that are available to them.[46] Accordingly, vision reports tend to be characterised by creative and consciously applied literary features such as careful structuring, thoughtful linguistic patterns and repetitions, poetic features as well as the use of metaphors, similes, allegories, quotations, allusion and symbolism.[47] Thus, the desire to convey the intensity of the perception will activate the artistic creativity of the visionary, which explains Rahner's conclusion that "Even in 'genuine' imaginative visions human powers are creatively at work."[48] This creative human contribution has been described expressively by Eddie Ensley as follows:

> Visions unleash our spontaneous religious imagination. Within each of us is a painter of sacred icons, a dramatist of inner mystery plays,

---

42 Lyons, "Envisioning Restoration," 74.

43 Werline ("Vision and Religious Experience," 7) sums up the difference between the two modes well: "Experience occupies the category of non-discursive knowledge, as opposed to discursive forms of apprehending or knowing, which tend to be more linear and logical and language based. The non-discursive inhabits the territory less visited by scholars."

44 Hildegard of Bingen, Letter 103R to Guibert of Gembloux (1175); cited in McGinn, *Christian Mysticism*, 333.

45 E.g. Rahner (*Visions and Prophecies*, 59) suggests that "a psychologically untrained, simple visionary in recollecting and relating his experience might (objectively speaking) overemphasize its imaginative element just because it is much easier to describe."

46 Drawing on the work of the 20th century scholar of Jewish mysticism, Gerson Scholem, Bernard McGinn (*Christian Mysticism*, 482) explains that in order to be understood, mystics must make use of the language and symbols of the tradition of their time; however, "the ineffable nature of the mystical sense of God also means that the inherited complex of symbols and language is never completely adequate to convey the message, and so mystics often attempt to stretch, transform, and deepen their tradition."

47 Lyons, "Envisioning Restoration," 74. By way of confirmation, in an analysis of medieval vision reports, Newman ("Medieval Visionary Culture," 3–4) concludes, "Most medieval vision texts, whether prose or verse, display at least some impulse toward artistic refinement."

48 Rahner, *Visions and Prophecies*, 72.

a poet of hallowed verse. At the touch of the eternal, that natural part of us forms metaphors and stories that become bridges. The paint buckets of the icon painter, the stories of the dramatist come from the realities of the world we live in – our culture, our lives, and our time. Our inner visionary storyteller, hidden in our unconscious, draws from all stories of our lives to form our visions.[49]

- *Theological framework*. In addition to the visionaries' creative touch, the report will also be affected by their theological training.[50] For example, even if one accepts that the basis of the Book of Revelation is a powerful visionary experience (or a series of experiences), it does not take more than a cursory inspection of the text to realise that the reporter of these experiences was well-versed in Jewish apocalyptic literature.[51] Drawing on Riceour's insights into the *a priory* conditions for human understanding, Christopher Rowland argues that visionaries make sense of visionary experiences through a framework of understanding that is already present in their cognition "at the level of the preconscious and precritical."[52] Thus, if the visionary's language proficiency is deeply rooted in biblical language, the report is bound to reflect this; indeed, talking about apocalyptic writers, Stone concludes that they "have to use the cultural language of their day and social context; *there is no other language for them to use*"[53] (emphasis in the original).

In Chapter 5 we shall address the potential vulnerabilities of vision that are related to the inevitably subjective and interpretive elements added to the vision report by the beholder, but we need to stress here that these vulnerabilities do not necessarily render vision reports inaccurate. Although the Scriptures do contain references to false prophets, who "speak visions from their own minds" (Jer 23:16), the authenticity of biblical prophecy was safeguarded by the fact that, as discussed earlier, divine vision was given only to a select group of God's trusted people. These hand-picked seers were steeped in scriptural tradition that was based on previous divine

---

49 Ensley, *Visions*, 113.
50 Rahner, *Visions and Prophecies*, 74. Proudfoot's (*Religious Experience*, 103) summary of Stephen Bradley's experience of the increase of his heart rate after a revival service (as described in detail in William James's *The Varieties of Religious Experience*), which led to Bradley's conversion, is equally true of a visionary experience: "Bradley, like so many prospective devotees before and since, could not understand his feelings in naturalistic terms. Religious symbols offered him an explanation that was compatible both with his experience and with his antecedent beliefs. He did not consider explanations involving Krishna, Zeus, or the Qur'an."
51 E.g. Rowland ("Visionary Experience," 43) highlights the close relationship between some parts of Revelation and prophetic texts such as Ezekiel and Daniel, although he stresses that the undoubted knowledge of these texts never manifests itself in explicit quotation.
52 Ibid., 45.
53 Stone, "Apocalyptic Vision," 179.

messages, and they used this as a conceptual framework within which the new messages could be interpreted. Thus, when we find parallels between certain imagery in Revelation and other apocalyptic literature, this may be viewed not as something that undermines the authenticity of the visionary experience presented in the text but rather as something that may actually *reinforce* it: the extraordinary imagery perceived by the seer John was mediated through a reliable theological frame of reference, namely, previously authenticated Jewish Scripture.[54]

Biblical vision reports as guided imagery

Sometimes the reader of Scripture cannot help feeling that an elaborate re-narration of a vision experience is partly aimed at evoking mental pictures in the audience so that they can re-live aspects of the vision through a form of transportation experience (discussed in Chapter 2) that we may call a "secondary" vision. A classic example of this sort of text is Isaiah's graphic images of "new heavens and a new earth" (65:17–25), with the following extract offering a good illustration of the expressive power of the text:

> No more shall there be in it
>   an infant that lives but a few days,
>   or an old person who does not live out a lifetime;
> for one who dies at a hundred years will be considered a youth,
>   and one who falls short of a hundred will be considered accursed.
> They shall build houses and inhabit them;
>   they shall plant vineyards and eat their fruit.
>
>   (vv. 20–21)

Since this "secondary" visionary experience is generated (either in the original audience or in contemporary readers of Scripture) by the vision report, the latter functions, in effect, as a form of "guided imagery" (as discussed in Chapter 2). There is, however, an important difference between this kind of directed imagery and the technique applied in psychotherapy, namely that, as Humphrey explains, "in the Jewish and Christian traditions, vision and words are typically conjoined, even while some aspects of the vision are left to make an imaginative rather than a cognitive impact."[55] Thus, she goes on, even while the reader is engaged by the "inherent mystery of the vision," the latter is scaffolded by "a clear interpretative word or directed

54 E.g. regarding Revelation, Rowland ("Visionary Experience," 43) submits: "John's vision draws on images that are familiar to us from elsewhere and in the history of interpretation have a fairly well-established meaning. Thus, the contribution of Dan 7 to the political symbolism of Rev 13 establishes a frame of reference that informs the sense we make of that chapter."
55 Humphrey, *Rhetoric of Vision*, 22.

context."[56] In other words, expressive descriptions of visionary scenes in the Bible can be considered almost like "guided imagery plus" in the sense that they contain a twofold message, pictorial and verbal, which makes them particularly effective according to Paivio's "dual coding theory" discussed in Chapter 1.

It needs to be stressed that despite their verbal underpinning, the reception of biblical texts characterised by this "guided imagery plus" element is different from the analytical reading of Scripture that focuses on, for example, doctrinal truths. Instead, as Rowland explains, such texts result in a "rather indirect relationship with the Scriptures in which the words become the catalyst for the exercise of imagination as text is taken up and infuses the imagination."[57] He calls this process of mixing verbal and imagery content "meditative imagination,"[58] and by means of illustration offers the interpretation of the vision in Ezekiel 1 (i.e. the prophet's visionary call, sometimes referred to as the "Throne Vision"), where "the meaning of the text may come about as the result of 'seeing again' what Ezekiel saw."[59] As he concludes, "Understanding, therefore, evokes a perception that pierces beyond the letter."[60] We shall see in Chapter 6 that this process of combining imagery and verbal content is at the heart of several established Christian practices of "cultivated vision," such as imaginative prayer, biblical meditation, "scripted vision" and even Ignatian spirituality in general.

Summary

This chapter has aimed at demonstrating the importance of vision as a biblical concept by showing that visionary experiences are frequently reported in the Scriptures and are involved in several key episodes of the biblical narrative. It was argued that biblical vision constitutes much more than mere pictures that are received by prophets: auditions, dreams, visitations and certain revelations may also belong to the broad domain of vision as defined in the first chapter, since they all involve receiving divine communication by utilising the faculty of mental imagery. In addition, there is good reason to extend the "visionary mode" to prophetic perception in general, which is borne out by the description of prophets as "seers" in Scripture as well as by the fact that the dominant verb of perception used in relation to prophecy is "to see" rather than "to hear" (i.e. a prophet "sees" the word of the Lord). Finally, it was shown that in certain special cases, "to see" and "to open one's eyes" are used in the Bible to refer to beholding divine insights that only one's inner senses could perceive. Most importantly in this respect,

---

56 Ibid.
57 Rowland, "Visionary Experience," 50.
58 Ibid.
59 Ibid., 56.
60 Ibid.

Paul's divine commission from Jesus was to "open the eyes" of the Gentiles so that they should turn from darkness to light.

Thus, examples of vision abound throughout the whole of the canon in various forms and contexts, and the sheer variety and number of vision-related episodes point to the profound role of vision in the very essence of the biblical narrative. In the final section of the chapter we addressed the question of how visionary experiences are related to the specific vision reports recorded in Scripture. It was argued that there are several confounding factors involved in the way a visionary experience is conveyed to readers in the written canon. To start with, the fact that these experiences are inherently individual and private adds an inevitable element of subjectivity to the report. This is further amplified by two additional factors: first, divine vision concerns an alternative reality that is outside the recipient's familiar domain or operation, which results in a certain amount of "fluidity" about how to make sense of these extraordinary experiences and how to best express their meaning to others; second, the visionary experiences are often nonverbal, involving a combination of varied modalities such as visual and auditory, which means that in order to produce a written vision report to be included in Scripture, it was necessary for the visionary to transform the experience into categories and structures of language – this could only be accomplished on the basis of the recipient's personal interpretation.

Given that there is no straightforward method of producing a written report of a divine vision, visionaries are compelled to rely on their individual creativity and theological training to describe what they have experienced in order to do full justice to their unique perception. As a result, vision reports invariably carry the mark of their recipients in one way or another. The validity of the specific reports recorded in the Scriptures was safeguarded by the careful selection of trusted recipients of divine revelation as well as by the biblical tradition that provided these recipients with a theological framework to interpret new messages truthfully. Yet, the Bible also contains repeated warnings about false prophets, which warrants some discussion of the potential vulnerabilities of vision in Chapter 5.

References

Arnold, William T. 1996. "Visions." In *Evangelical Dictionary of Biblical Theology*, edited by Walter A. Elwell, 802–3. Grand Rapids, MI: Baker Books.

Ashley, Timothy R. 1993. *The Book of Numbers*. New International Commentary on the Old Testament. Grand Rapids, MI: Eerdmans.

Aune, David E. 1988a. "Ecstasy." In *The International Standard Bible Encyclopedia, Revised*, edited by Geoffrey W. Bromiley, 14–16. Grand Rapids, MI: Eerdmans.

Aune, David E. 1988b. "Vision." In *The International Standard Bible Encyclopedia, Revised*, edited by Geoffrey W. Bromiley, 993–94. Grand Rapids, MI: Eerdmans.

Boyd, Gregory A. 2004. *Seeing Is Believing: Experience Jesus through Imaginative Prayer*. Grand Rapids, MI: Baker Books.

Braun, Roddy. 1986. *1 Chronicles*. Word Biblical Commentary. Dallas, TX: Word Books.

Brueggemann, Walter. 1997. *Theology of the Old Testament: Testimony, Dispute, Advocacy*. Minneapolis, MN: Fortress.

Brueggemann, Walter. 2001. *The Prophetic Imagination*. 2nd ed. Minneapolis, MN: Fortress.

Dunn, James D. G. 1997. "Biblical Concepts of Revelation." In *Divine Revelation*, edited by Paul Avis, 1–22. Eugene, OR: Wipf and Stock.

Ensley, Eddie. 2000. *Visions: The Soul's Path to the Sacred*. Chicago: Loyola Press.

Everts, Janet Meyer. 1992. "Dreams in the New Testament and Greco-Roman Literature." In *The Anchor Bible Dictionary*, edited by David Noel Freedman, 231–31. New York: Doubleday.

Groeschel, Benedict J. 1993. *A Still, Small Voice: A Practical Guide on Reported Revelations*. San Francisco: Ignatius.

Hanson, John S. 1980. "Dreams and Visions in the Graeco-Roman World and Early Christianity." In *Aufstieg und Niedergang der Römischen Welt, Part Ii*, edited by Hildegard Temporini and Wolfgang Haase, 1395–427. Berlin: Walter de Gruyter.

Hayes, Elizabeth R., and Lena-Sofia Tiemeyer, eds. 2014. *"I Lifted My Eyes and Saw": Reading Dream and Vision Reports in the Hebrew Bible*. London: Bloomsbury T&T Clark.

Humphrey, Edith M. 2007. *And I Turned to See the Voice: The Rhetoric of Vision in the New Testament*. Grand Rapids, MI: Baker Academic.

James, William. 1917. *The Varieties of Religious Experience a Study in Human Nature*. New York: Longmans, Green, and Co.

Lyons, Michael A. 2014. "Envisioning Restoration: Innovations in Ezekiel 40–48." In *"I Lifted My Eyes and Saw": Reading Dream and Vision Reports in the Hebrew Bible*, edited by Elizabeth R. Hayes and Lena-Sofia Tiemeyer, 71–83. London: Bloomsbury T&T Clark.

Macalister, Alex. 1915. "Trance." In *International Standard Bible Encyclopaedia* edited by James Orr, John L. Nuelsen, Edgar Y. Mullins and Morris O. Evans. 3005. Chicago: Howard-Severance.

Martin, Ralph P. 2014. *2 Corinthians*. Word Biblical Commentary 40. 2nd ed. Grand Rapids, MI: Zondervan.

McGinn, Bernard. 2006. *The Essential Writings of Christian Mysticism*. New York: Modern Library.

Miller, John B. F. 2007. *Convinced That God Had Called Us: Dreams, Visions and the Perception of God's Will in Luke-Acts*. Leiden: Brill.

Miller, John B. F. 2013. "Dreams and Visions." In *Dictionary of Jesus and the Gospels; Second Edition* edited by Joel B. Green, Jeannine K. Brown and Norman Perrin, 216–18. Downers Grove, IL: IVP Academic.

Newman, Barbara. 2005. "What Did It Mean to Say "I Saw"? The Clash between Theory and Practice in Medieval Visionary Culture." *Speculum* 80, no. 1: 1–43.

Packer, J. I. 1996. "Revelation." In *New Bible Dictionary*, edited by I. Howard Marshall, A. R. Millard, J. I. Packer and D. J. Wiseman, 1014–16. Downers Grove, IL: InterVarsity Press.

Paul, Ian. 2018. *Revelation*. London: Inter-Varsity Press.

Proudfoot, Wayne. 1985. *Religious Experience*. Berkeley, CA: University of California Press.

Rahner, Karl. 1963. *Visions and Prophecies*. Translated by Charles H. Henkey and Richard Strachan. Freiburg: Herder.

Roberts, Ronald D. 2016. "Dream." In *The Lexham Bible Dictionary*, edited by John D. Barry, David Bomar, Derek R. Brown, Rachel Klippenstein, Douglas Mangum, Carrie Sinclair Wolcott, Lazarus Wentz, Elliot Ritzema and Wendy Widder. Bellingham, WA: Lexham Press.

Rowland, Christopher (with Patricia Gibbons, and Vicente Dobroruka). 2006. "Visionary Experience in Ancient Judaism and Christianity." In *Paradise Now: Essays on Early Jewish and Christian Mysticism*, edited by April D. DeConick, 41–56. Atlanta, GA: Society of Biblical Literature.

Ryken, Leland, James C. Wilhoit, and Tremper III Longman. 1998. "Dreams, Visions." In *Dictionary of Biblical Imagery*, 217–19. Downers Grove, IL: InterVarsity Press.

Scalise, Pamela. 2014. "Vision Beyond the Visions in Jeremiah." In *"I Lifted My Eyes and Saw": Reading Dream and Vision Reports in the Hebrew Bible*, edited by Elizabeth R. Hayes and Lena-Sofia Tiemeyer, 47–58. London: Bloomsbury T&T Clark.

Silva, Moisés, ed. 2014. *NIDNTTE (New International Dictionary of New Testament Theology and Exegesis)*. 2nd ed. Grand Rapids, MI: Zondervan.

Stead, Michael R. 2012. "Visions, Prophetic." In *Dictionary of the Old Testament: Prophets*, edited by Mark J. Boda and Gordon J. McConville, 818–26. Downers Grove, IL: IVP Academic.

Stone, Michael E. 2003. "A Reconsideration of Apocalyptic Visions." *Harvard Theological Review* 96, no. 2: 167–80.

Thrall, Margaret E. 1994. *A Critical and Exegetical Commentary on the Second Epistle of the Corinthians*. International Critical Commentary. Vol. 1, London: T & T Clark.

Warfield, Benjamin B. 1915. "Revelation." In *The International Standard Bible Encyclopaedia*, edited by J. Orr, J. L. Nuelsen, E. Y. Mullins and M. O. Evans, 2573–82. Chicago: The Howard-Severance Company.

Werline, Rodney A. 2014. "Assessing the Prophetic Vision and Dream Texts for Insights into Religious Experience." In *"I Lifted My Eyes and Saw": Reading Dream and Vision Reports in the Hebrew Bible*, edited by Elizabeth R. Hayes and Lena-Sofia Tiemeyer, 1–15. London: Bloomsbury T&T Clark.

Williams, Stephen N. 2005. "Revelation." In *Dictionary for Theological Interpretation of the Bible*, edited by Kevin J. Vanhoozer, 678–80. London: SPCK.

4   The essence of biblical vision

The discussion in the previous chapter extended the scope of the notion of biblical vision beyond the narrow understanding of prophets receiving divinely inspired visual imagery. This, however, raises the question of what the various forms of imagery share in common as the essence of biblical vision. The current chapter highlights two central aspects in this respect, one related to the general *function* of vision, the other to its specific *purpose*. Regarding the former, it will be proposed that visionary experiences in the Bible predominantly concern *divine communication* between the heavenly and the earthly realms, and regarding the latter, that most of these communications have a *motivational purpose*, understood in a broad sense. This being the case, the essence of biblical vision will be presented as constituting a vehicle for God's interventions in human affairs in order to facilitate the progressive transformation of humans into citizens of the kingdom of God.

Vision as the channel of divine communication

All the different types of vision in the Scriptures are consistent in one crucial aspect: they concern a juncture of the celestial and human spheres, a crossing that is described by different scholars as "an irruption of the divine presence into human affairs,"[1] "the intersection of the heavenly and earthly realms in some way,"[2] "a real intervention and influence from the other world"[3] or simply "an invasion from above."[4] That is, visionary experiences reported in the Scriptures are platforms for communication between heaven and earth, making vision the primary interface in the Bible between the spiritual and material spheres that humans can tune into in order to catch glimpses of non-material reality and to receive celestial messages. A further commonality of the various vision reports in the Bible is that the celestial messages predominantly originate from, or are authorised by,

1 Miller, *Dreams and Visions in Luke-Acts*, 7.
2 Guthrie, *2 Corinthians*, 577.
3 Rahner, *Visions and Prophecies*, 7.
4 Derek Tidball, personal communication.

God[5] – Jeremiah 23:16, for example, describes false prophets as ones who "speak visions . . . not from the mouth of the LORD," which indicates that a true biblical vision has to come from God.

The direct link between divine communication and prophetic vision is also underlined in Amos 3:8, where prophecy is depicted as being just as irresistible as the fearful reaction when a lion roars: "The lion has roared; who will not fear? The Lord God has spoken; who can but prophesy?" Douglas Stuart highlights a similar inevitability[6] expressed by the Apostle Paul in 1 Corinthians with regard to acting upon the vision he received[7] by preaching the gospel: "an obligation is laid on me, and woe to me if I do not proclaim the gospel!" Further confirmation of the divine origins of a true biblical vision is offered by the first two verses of Hebrews: after declaring that "Long ago God spoke to our ancestors in many and various ways by the prophets" (1:1), the text continues, "but in these last days he has spoken to us by a Son" (v. 2). Indeed, during the public ministry of Jesus (i.e. between his baptism and Calvary), the Gospels mention only one single instance of vision, the Transfiguration (Matt 17:9). The absence of any further visions during the unique period when God could communicate with humans directly though his Son confirms that the essence of biblical vision was to function as the channel of divine communication, because, as Janet Everts rightly points out in the *Anchor Bible Dictionary*, "Dreams and visions are not necessary when God chooses to reveal himself in such a direct and unequivocal way."[8] After all, as Colossians 1:15 proclaims, Jesus is "the image of the invisible God," that is, divine vision materialised.

The understanding that the essence of vision is centred around divine communication is also supported by a key oracle in Numbers 12:6–8; because this passage includes a rare instance when the Scriptures offer explicit teaching on the nature of visionary communication, it will be analysed in a separate section below, to be followed by the examination of two related themes: the role of the Holy Spirit in facilitating the reception of vision as well as the connection of vision to being created in God's image and the theological concept of the "inner man."

An oracle on divine communication (Numbers 12:6–8)

In Numbers 12 we read that Aaron and Miriam challenged Moses's authority as a leader, and v. 2 reveals that a key element of their argument concerned

---

5 Although, as we shall see in Chapter 5 when discussing the vulnerability of vision, the visionary mode can also be utilised by spiritual forces with an agenda other than God's, but this is a very rare occurrence in the Scriptures.
6 Stuart, *Hosea – Jonah*, 325–326.
7 See Gal 1:11.
8 Everts, "Dreams," 231. This notion might also underlie what Jesus said to the disciples: "many prophets and righteous people longed to see what you see, but did not see it, and to hear what you hear, but did not hear it" (Matt 13:17; see also Luke 10:24).

hearing from God: "Has the Lord spoken only through Moses? Has he not spoken through us also?" According to the narrative, this challenge prompted God to summon Moses, Aaron and Miriam to the tabernacle in order to explain to them some ground rules about divine communication:

> When there are prophets among you,
>   I the Lord make myself known to them in visions;
>   I speak to them in dreams.
> Not so with my servant Moses;
>   he is entrusted with all my house.
> With him I speak face to face – clearly, not in riddles;
>   and he beholds the form of the Lord.
>
> (Num 12:6–8)

The first important point to consider in the passage is the phrase "face to face" in v. 8. The original Hebrew text says "mouth to mouth" and the common translation into "face to face" (e.g. by the NRSV and NIV) is partly due to the parallel description of God knowing Moses "face to face" in Deuteronomy 34:10 and especially the statement in Exodus 33:11: "Thus the Lord used to speak to Moses face to face, as one speaks to a friend." However, in these latter cases the Hebrew original does indeed use the word "face," unlike in Numbers 12:8, where the phrase "mouth to mouth" is used as a single occurrence in the Bible.[9] Of course, speaking to someone "mouth to mouth" involves an interlocutor who faces the speaker, so "mouth to mouth" does not contradict "face to face"; rather, it offers a *more specific* meaning, as if to be more precise about the nature of the communication. Such precision is, in fact, in line with the overall purpose of God's oracle, namely to clarify the issue of how he communicated with humans. The question, then, is what this more specific meaning refers to? From a linguistic point of view, the obvious meaning of "mouth to mouth communication" is *verbal communication*, that is communication mostly through words. Does this meaning seem right and relevant in this passage? Not if the interpretation of the text centres around the theme of authority challenge (which is probably why both the NRSV and the NIV paraphrased it to "face to face"); however, within the framework of our current discussion centred around the nature of vision, such a specification makes perfect sense. From this perspective, the oracle in effect states that the primary distinction between God's communication with prophets and Moses lies in the *mode of communication*: straightforward verbal messages (Moses) versus visions, dreams and riddles (prophets).

What is the significance of this distinction? From a communication point of view, the contrast denotes a major difference with respect to the

---

9 Dozeman, *Book of Numbers,* 110.

comprehensibility of the message: the common feature of visions/dreams and riddles (i.e. the mode of communication associated with the prophets) is that they do not convey a plain verbal message but rather an enriched version of it by adding imagery or by requiring extra cognitive engagement (i.e. to decipher a riddle). These added elements increase the power of the message content – or as is sometimes referred to in linguistics, the "illocutionary force" of the utterance – which in turn ensures that the message is less likely misunderstood and will thus invoke the expected response.[10] Accordingly, in contrast to the use of unmediated verbal communication with his trusted servant Moses,[11] God relied, in effect, on an *enhanced* mode of communication with other humans to safeguard the comprehension of his intended message.[12] Such a concern with human understanding is fully consistent with the fact that before Pentecost, visions and dreams were given only to a select few – the prophets – in order to ensure that God's visionary message would be appropriately interpreted and conveyed to others. God's unique relationship of trust in Moses is also reflected in v. 7, where God declares about him that "he is entrusted with all my house."[13]

In sum, the main lesson of the Numbers passage for the current discussion is twofold: first, Aaron's and Miriam's challenge revealed that the status of God's servants was related to their being recipients of divine communication. Indeed, Thomas Dozeman is right in pointing out that the fact that it was Aaron and Miriam who challenged Moses may not merely be due to the family ties with him but also to the fact that besides Abraham they are the only other characters called "prophets" in the entire Pentateuch (in Exod 7:1 and 15:20, respectively).[14] Second and more importantly, God declared that his means of communication with humans will involve the channel of *mental*

10 Indeed, an important tenet of speech act theory is that the strength of the illocutionary force of an utterance is the function of its "mode of achievement," that is, the manner in which the message is delivered, and we have seen in the first chapters (e.g. when discussing Paivio's dual coding theory) that the combination of verbal and imagery-based processing results in augmented cognitive effectiveness due to the added experiential content.

11 Having said that, Num 12:8 states that Moses "beholds the form of the Lord," which indicates that some form of visionary channel still existed between him and God. Wenham (*Numbers*, 127) explains that the Hebrew word for "form" (*tĕmûnâ*) "is used of visual representations, pictures or images, of earthly and heavenly beings (Exod. 20:4). . . . Thus, although Moses enjoyed a much closer relationship with God than any ordinary prophet, he saw only God's form, not the very being of God." This, however, is not unexpected, given that "God is spirit" (John 4:24).

12 We may recall at this point that Job only understood God's message when his "seeing" complemented his "hearing" ("I had heard of you by the hearing of the ear, but now my eye sees you; therefore I despise myself, and repent in dust and ashes"; Job 42:5–6); in contrast, Moses's special status was marked by the fact that he did not need the "seeing" aspect to understand God.

13 Although not directly related to this issue, it is noteworthy that at the Transfiguration one of the people to whom the transfigured (i.e. deified) Christ spoke was Moses, who could speak to God directly, and the other was Elijah, who was raptured alive from the earth by God, presumably to have a direct relationship with him.

14 Dozeman, *Book of Numbers*, 109.

imagery mediated by prophets, which affirms the fact that visions in the Bible function as an interface between the Creator and his people.

The theological understanding of biblical vision as a channel of divine communication goes back as far as the church fathers; for example, Veerle Fraeters reports that in his influential writings, Saint Gregory the Great (c. 540–604) repeatedly underlined the importance of spiritual vision, stating that the "eyes of the heart" (*cordis oculis*) – or as he sometimes called them, the "eyes of the mind" (*mentis oculis*) – are the organ with which the human mind can apprehend God's message.[15] In modern times, Paul Avis amongst others has argued in a similar vein, stating that "divine revelation is given above all (though certainly not exclusively) in modes that are addressed to the human imagination, rather than to any other faculty (such as the analytical reason or the moral conscience)."[16] Gregory Boyd also submits that "God's ordinary mode of communication, both in biblical times and today, is to speak and appear to those who have the spiritual capacity to hear and see spiritual realities."[17]

The role of the Holy Spirit in facilitating the reception of vision

In his overview of vision in the Bible, Arnold concludes that the "extensive use of the term in nearly all the Old Testament prophets implies that visions were a normal medium for receiving the divine word,"[18] and the discussion in the previous section has been consistent with this claim. Yet, this may not be the complete picture, because the Scriptures highlight one further element in the divine communication process (besides vision) that is required for receiving God's messages: the involvement of the Holy Spirit. This was first expressed by Moses himself in his yearning, "Would that all the Lord's people were prophets, and that the Lord would put his spirit on them!" (Num 11:29), and elsewhere in the Scriptures we find several explicit references to the Spirit's involvement in prophets perceiving divine messages. For example, Ezekiel 2:2 states, "As he [a voice in Ezekiel's vision] spoke, the Spirit came into me and raised me to my feet, and I heard him speaking to me" (NIV; see also 3:24; 11:5), and in a passage in Joel that will be further explored in a separate section, the Spirit's role in enabling a visionary experience is emphasised twice:

> And afterward,
>   I will *pour out my Spirit* on all people.
> Your sons and daughters will prophesy,
>   your old men will dream dreams,
>   your young men will see visions.

15 Fraeters, "Vision/Vision," 179.
16 Avis, *God and the Creative Imagination*, 3.
17 Boyd, *Seeing Is Believing*, 84.
18 Arnold, "Visions," 802–803.

> Even on my servants, both men and women,
>   I will *pour out my Spirit* in those days.
> I will show wonders in the heavens
>   and on the earth.
>   (Joel 2:28–30; NIV, emphasis added)

We shall see later that Peter cited this passage in his speech at Pentecost to the bewildered crowd and then reiterated the Spirit's role in an explicit reference: "he [Jesus] has poured out[19] this that you both see and hear" (Acts 2:33). The connection between vision and the Spirit is further highlighted in 2 Peter 1:20, where we read that "no prophecy ever came by human will, but men and women moved by the Holy Spirit spoke from God." In a similar vein, the seer John starts reporting his majestic vision at the beginning of Revelation by stating, "I was in the Spirit, and I heard behind me a loud voice like a trumpet, which said: 'Write on a scroll what you see . . .'" (1:10–11; NIV). Interestingly, sometimes the Spirit's involvement is emphasised by actually equating him with the agency of the visionary message, as is done, for example in Acts 10:19: "While Peter was still thinking about the vision, the Spirit said to him, 'Look, three men are searching for you. . . .'"[20]

We may thus conclude that, similar to how John 4:24 declares that "God is spirit, and his worshipers must worship in the Spirit and in truth" (NIV), the perception of God's communication also requires a Spirit-filled mindset. As Gregory Boyd sums up, "imagination, when guided by the Holy Spirit and submitted to the authority of Scripture, is our main receptor to the spiritual world."[21] This is in harmony with 1 Corinthians 2:9–10: "as is written, 'What no eye has seen, nor ear heard, nor the human heart conceived, what God has prepared for those who love him' – these things God has revealed to us through the Spirit."

"Created in his image . . ." and the "inner man"

It was mentioned in the Introduction that Augustine of Hippo firmly believed in the spiritual nature of vision, as shown, for example, by his contention that "there is a kind of spiritual element in us where the likenesses of bodily things [i.e. visions] are formed."[22] In view of the previous discussion that

---

19 The same verb (*ekcheō*) is used here as in the reciting of the Joel prophecy in Acts 2:17 ("I will pour out my Spirit upon all flesh"), thereby creating a conscious link; see e.g. Bock, *Acts*, 131.
20 Miller (*Dreams and Visions in Luke-Acts*, 14) highlights in this respect the related fact that in Acts 10 we read about Cornelius that he "had a vision in which he clearly saw an angel of God" (v. 3) who told him to go send men to Joppa to invite Peter (v. 5); Peter, however, is told by the Spirit about the men searching for him that "I have sent them" (v. 20), thereby coalescing the actions of the Spirit with those of the angel in the vision.
21 Boyd, *Seeing Is Believing*, 16.
22 Augustine, *On the Literal Meaning of Genesis*, 12.49 (p. 490).

indicated that this "spiritual element in us" is predominantly associated in the Bible with the ability to participate in divine communication, it may not be unreasonable to assume that when God created humans "in his image" (Gen 1:27), equipping them with the faculty of vision was a core aspect of this "image." This point was also made in the classic *International Standard Bible Encyclopaedia* in 1915, where Charles Stuart concluded:

> Whether man was made this way in order that God might communicate with him through dreams and visions is hardly worth debating; if the records of human life, in the Bible and out of it, are to be trusted at all, there is nothing better certified than that God has communicated with man in this way (Ps 89:19; Prov 29:18; cf. Am 8:11, 12; Hos 12:10).[23]

Indeed, recognising that humans have a dual sensory system (i.e. external and internal) and linking the internal senses to the perception of glimpses of transcendent reality and especially to receiving direct communications from the heavenly sphere has had a long history in theology. In Book XII of *The Literal Meaning of Genesis*, Augustine referred to the two sets of senses as (a) "corporeal vision" (*visio corporalis*), which is the vision "with which we see heaven and earth and everything in them that is visible to our eyes," and (b) "spiritual vision" (*visio spiritualis*), "by which absent bodies are thought about in a bodily fashion."[24] He further explains the latter as follows:

> when we are standing in the dark, we can think about the sky and the earth and all the things we can see in them; we are not seeing anything with the eyes in our heads, but we are looking all the same at bodily images with the spirit, whether they be true ones like the bodies we have seen and retained the memory of, or fictitious ones the imagination may have constructed.[25]

This conceptualisation, which was widely shared by church fathers and theologians across the Christian spectrum and which also had a profound impact on subsequent mysticism,[26] is noteworthy for its sophistication: it is remarkable that the insights Augustine discerned without having any empirical research base are fully consistent with the relevant tenets proposed by modern neuroscience.

---

23 Stuart, "Vision," 3057.
24 Augustine, *On the Literal Meaning of Genesis*, 12.15 (p. 470). Augustine also distinguished a third, "intellectual vision," which "touches on things which do not have any images," but as this category does not contain any actual imagery element, it will not be covered in the current discussion.
25 Ibid., 470.
26 For overviews, see e.g. Dailey, "The Body and Its Senses," 264; Fraeters, "Vision/Vision," 178–179; Harrison, "Spiritual Senses," 768; Wright, "Mysticism," 579.

The twofold sensory endowment of human beings has also been connected to the dichotomy of the "inner man" versus the "outer man" that is presented in three New Testament epistles (Rom 7:22; 2 Cor 4:16; Eph 3:16). Hans Urs von Balthasar explains that Origen was the first theologian to construct a doctrine of the "double human being,"[27] explicitly linking the inner/outer men to two types of seeing,[28] and in his *Commentary on the Epistle to the Romans*, Origen submits that the inner man was "made in the image of God" and the outer man was "formed from the mud of the earth."[29]

The broadening of the reception of divine communication after Pentecost

We gain further insight into the essence of biblical vision when we consider how the initial circle of partakers in divine communication was extended later in the biblical story. According to God's declaration in Numbers (discussed above), the potential recipients of divine vision were restricted to a select group of intermediaries, called the "prophets." It was argued earlier that this limitation served to ensure that the divine messages were fully comprehended, and then correctly interpreted and enacted. It is against this background that the first two verses of an oracle in Joel 2 (28–3:8) concerning a momentous future event gain special significance, as they predict a dramatic broadening of the reception of divine communication:

> Then afterward
>   I will pour out my spirit on all flesh;
> your sons and your daughters shall prophesy,
>   your old men shall dream dreams,
>   and your young men shall see visions.
> Even on the male and female slaves,
>   in those days, I will pour out my spirit.
>
>   (vv. 28–29)

Given the fact that, as seen in the analysis of the passage in Numbers 12 earlier, the status of God's servants was directly related to their being recipients of divine communication, Joel's prophecy foreshadowed a new social order amongst God's human stewards. According to the oracle, the transformation would affect the whole spectrum of society, since the traditional

---

27 von Balthasar, *Origen*, 218. We should note, however, that as Dailey ("The Body and Its Senses," 264) rightly points out, the notion of an inner human being was also present in Hellenic thought, associated with the *nous* (mind) or *psyche* (the soul) as parts of human existence prevailing in the afterlife.
28 Ibid., 221–222.
29 Origen, *Commentary on the Epistle to the Romans*, II, 13, 34.

markers of social standing (age, gender, social status) were to be overridden by the outpouring of the Spirit and the "democratisation" of vision.[30] It is noteworthy that the oracle also promised the fulfilment of Moses's aspiration in Numbers 11:29 – "Would that all the Lord's people were prophets, that the Lord would put his spirit upon them" – because when the predicted events were to happen, all God's people would become, in effect, prophets.[31] Finally, what makes this remarkable oracle even more significant for our current discussion is that the oracle was declared to have come true by the Apostle Peter at Pentecost, thereby linking vision directly to one of the main milestones in the history of Christianity.

Pentecost and its consequences

Pentecost offers a striking example in the biblical corpus of the actual fulfilment of a significant earlier prophetic vision, foretold in Joel's oracle mentioned earlier. According to the description in Acts 2, the dramatic events that accompanied the Spirit's powerful move in Jerusalem required an immediate interpretation for the bewildered crowd, and the Apostle Peter responded to this need by delivering the first Christian sermon recorded in the Bible. In this, quite remarkably, he began by quoting at length Joel's prophecy (Acts 2:17–21), and Howard Marshall explains that by starting his citation with "In the last days . . ." (v. 17) instead of "Then afterward . . ." (Joel 2:28), Peter implies that "his hearers are now living in the last days. God's final act of salvation has begun to take place."[32] In other words, in Peter's description of "the last days," the reception of dreams and visions come right at the beginning as a direct correlate with the outpouring of the Holy Spirit, thereby reiterating Joel's vision of having a forthcoming new intimacy with God for "everyone who calls on the name of the Lord" (Acts 2:21), irrespective of one's gender, age and outward status.

We find a good illustration of the inclusive nature of this change in Acts 9:10, concerning the vision that Ananias received about Paul's conversion: "Now there was a disciple in Damascus named Ananias. The Lord said to him in a vision, 'Ananias.' He answered, 'Here I am, Lord.'" What is important about this passage for the current discussion is that Ananias was neither described as a prophet nor a church/community leader, but merely as a "devout man according to the law and well spoken of by all the Jews

---

30 See, e.g. Baker, *Joel, Obadiah, Malachi,* 108. Some scholars argue that the pronouns "*your* sons and *your* daughters" signify that the oracle concerns only the people of Israel, which was strictly speaking true at Pentecost, but this restriction loses its relevance in view of the fact that Paul explains in Rom 11:7 that Gentile believers are grafted onto the rootstock of the Israelites, thereby creating continuity. This continuity was indeed evidenced by the "Gentile Pentecost" in Acts 10:44–46.

31 See e.g. Hubbard, *Joel and Amos,* 73.

32 Marshall, *Acts,* 78.

living there" (Acts 22:12); yet, in the post-Pentecostal era he could become a central figure in a divinely orchestrated scenario that replicated the calling of the prophet Samuel in the Old Testament (1 Sam 3:4): "Then the Lord called, 'Samuel! Samuel!' and he said, 'Here I am!'"

The activation of the human faculty of vision through the release of the Holy Spirit was to play a vital role in the advancement of Christianity, as it enabled believers to receive private revelations from God. In his "Farewell Discourse" (John 14–17), Jesus declared that there were certain things that humanity was not ready to "bear" at that time and therefore further guidance would come from future prophecies/visions through the Holy Spirit: "I still have many things to say to you, but you cannot bear them now. When the Spirit of truth comes, he will guide you into all the truth . . . and he will declare to you the things that are to come" (16:12–13). The Spirit-filled endowment of beholding God's vision that was made widely available at Pentecost marked the beginning of the realisation of these promises, and the New Testament contains several vision reports that bear witness to the profound impact of the divine messages thus received. We shall conclude this chapter by surveying some of the most important biblical examples in this respect.

Examples of vision in the New Testament

As pointed out earlier, no divine vision of any kind is mentioned in the New Testament during Jesus' adult ministry apart from the Transfiguration, but we do find in Matthew's Gospel a handful of mentions of vision related to Jesus' infancy: the wise men from the East are warned in a dream not to return to Herod (2:12); the Lord's angel appears in a dream to Joseph telling him to flee to Egypt (2:13); the Lord's angel tells Joseph to return to Israel (2:19); and Joseph is warned not to settle in Judea but in Galilee (2:22). Then, after Jesus' death, several people saw an angel (or two angels) at Jesus' tomb (Matt 28:4–5; Mark 16:5; Luke 24:4), and before his ascension, Jesus appeared to many people, although it is uncertain whether seeing the resurrected Son of God counts as a vision or not. In any case, the visionary experiences related to Jesus are best kept separate as a unique category, as they concern the Son of God, who himself is "the image of the invisible God" (Col 1:15).

After the "democratisation" of vision at Pentecost, visionary experiences play a decisive role in the narrative of Acts, and David deSilva concludes that a revelation from the Holy Spirit is linked to each new development in the early church.[33] To illustrate the significance of the divine guidance – or as

---

33 deSilva, "Visions," 1195. He lists Philip's evangelising (Acts 8:26, 39–40), Paul's conversion and reception into the church by Ananias (Acts 9:3–17), Paul's timely departure from Jerusalem and reorientation towards a Gentile mission (Acts 22:17–21), Peter's preaching to the household of the Gentile Cornelius (Acts 10:3–6, 9–16), Paul and Barnabas's

deSilva calls it, "God's orchestration of the Christian movement"[34] – let us consider the visions of the two leading NT apostles, Peter and Paul. Peter's most momentous visionary experience occurs in a sequence of a "paired vision": first the Roman centurion Cornelius is told in a vision by an angel of the Lord to send men to fetch Peter (Acts 10:3–6), then Peter has a vision on the rooftop of his house about eating unclean animals (vv. 9–13) – and when he is reluctant to accept the message, the image is repeated three times (vv. 14–16) – followed by the Spirit's instruction that he should go with Cornelius's men who has just arrived at his home (vv. 19–20). This complex visionary sequence led to what is sometimes referred to as the "Gentile Pentecost" (vv. 44–48; i.e. when the Spirit fell powerfully on Gentile believers in Cornelius's house), resulting ultimately in the decision taken at the Council of Jerusalem to accept Gentiles into the emerging Christian church (15:6–21). Presumably due to the magnitude of the events, the visionary elements are emphasised in the narrative by multiple repetitions: Cornelius's vision is related as many as four times (Acts 10:3–6, 22, 30–32; 11:13–14) and Peter's three times (Acts 10:9–20, 28–29; 11:4–12), leaving absolutely no doubt in the audience about the crucial part that divine vision played in orchestrating these happenings.

Paul's dramatic visionary experience[35] on the road to Damascus is also recounted three times in the Scriptures (Acts 9:3–9; 22:6–11; 26:12–18) and it, too, is followed by a "paired vision," with the added twist that the second vision is reported as part of the first, when Ananias is told in a vision about Paul having a vision about him:

> The Lord said to him in a vision, "Ananias." He answered, "Here I am, Lord." The Lord said to him, "Get up and go to the street called Straight, and at the house of Judas look for a man of Tarsus named Saul. At this moment he is praying, and he has seen in a vision a man named Ananias come in and lay his hands on him so that he might regain his sight."
>
> (Acts 9:10–12)

Paul's story offers an intriguing interaction of physical and spiritual sight, because after he experienced divine vision on the road to Damascus, he was blinded and remained sightless for three days. Yet, Edith Humphrey is right

---

commission (Acts 13:2), Paul and Barnabas's mission to Macedonia (Acts 16:6–10), Paul's preaching in Corinth (Acts 18:9–10), Paul's imprisonment and trial (Acts 20:23) and Paul's testimony in Rome (Acts 23:11; 27:23–24).

34 Ibid.

35 One may wonder whether this experience was in fact visionary in nature as there was no "visual" element reported besides exposure to bright light (see e.g. Humphrey, *Rhetoric of Vision*, 83–84). However, it was argued in Chapter 1 that auditions count as vision and Paul also reports Jesus telling him about "things in which you have seen me and to those in which I will appear to you" (Acts 26:16).

that "Ironically, it is in being blinded that Saul really begins to see. It is in his state of blindness that he is brought to pray and sees in a vision his cure."[36] The reason for the blind period is not stated in the Scriptures, but if we consider the neuroscientific background of vision (i.e. the joint cerebral areas for processing physical sight and mental imagery), it may be argued that an important consequence of Paul's physical blindness was that for three days physical sight did not override the visionary mode in him. This allowed sufficient time for the visionary stimuli to exercise their profound transformational impact. Another possible reason for the temporary blindness and the subsequent miraculous recovery may have been to offer Paul compelling evidence about the authenticity of the divine vision he had received, which would be consistent with the occurrence of the "paired vision," which also played a crucial part in convincing Peter of the authenticity of the visionary message he received.

There are also clear indications in the text that the visionary experience on the road to Damascus was to be followed by further visions: in Ananias's vision the Lord tells him that "I myself will *show* him how much he must suffer for the sake of my name" (Acts 9:16; emphasis added), and Paul also reports Jesus telling him to "testify to the things in which you have seen me and to those in which *I will appear to you*" (26:16; emphasis added). Consistent with this, in his letter to the Galatians, Paul declares about the gospel he proclaimed that it was "not of human origin; for I did not receive it from a human source, nor was I taught it, but I received it through a *revelation* of Jesus Christ" (1:11; emphasis added). The Scriptures report several further visions experienced by Paul, with one containing the man of Macedonia calling him in a dream (Acts 16:9), which resulted in the gospel reaching Europe, and in 2 Corinthians Paul also describes a visionary journey up to the third heaven (2 Cor 12:2–4).

The motivational purpose of biblical vision

Although references to vision are numerous in the Bible and visionary experiences occur in varied forms, commentators have proposed relatively few specific purposes that these visions were intended to serve, and most of these are connected with *motivation* in one way or another. "Motivation" as a technical term is used in psychology to explain three main facets of human behaviour: *why* people decide to do something, *how long* they are willing to sustain the activity and *how hard* they are going to pursue it – or, in psychological terms, the *choice* of a particular action, the *persistence* with it and the *effort* expended on it.[37] As will be illustrated below, we find instances of vision in the Bible representing each of these three functions.

---

36 Ibid., 87.
37 See e.g. Dörnyei and Ushioda, *Teaching and Researching Motivation*, 4.

Regarding the *choice of action*, biblical characters are often instructed in visions or dreams about what they should or should not do, ranging from God sending Jacob to Egypt in a vision of the night (Gen 46:2–4) to several message dreams Joseph (Mary's husband) received concerning the infant Jesus (Matt 1:20–2:22) mentioned earlier. Acts 26:15–16 offers a particularly clear example of a motivational directive, Paul's commissioning by Jesus: "I am Jesus . . . I have appeared to you for this purpose, to appoint you to serve and testify to the things in which you have seen me and to those in which I will appear to you." The normative power of this directive was evidenced in 1 Corinthians 9:16, where Paul states that "an obligation is laid on me, and woe to me if I do not proclaim the gospel!" and Acts 26:19 recounts Paul telling King Agrippa that he was "not disobedient to the heavenly vision."

A second group of visionary experience is aimed at encouraging the recipients and thus enhancing their *effort* and *persistence*, consistent with Paul's explanation of the main functions of genuine prophecy in 1 Corinthians 14:3: "those who prophesy speak to other people for their upbuilding and encouragement and consolation." A classic example of an encouraging message fostering perseverance is offered by Paul in a speech to the sailors on his way to Rome before the shipwreck at Malta:

> I urge you now to keep up your courage, for there will be no loss of life among you, but only of the ship. For last night there stood by me an angel of the God to whom I belong and whom I worship, and he said, "Do not be afraid, Paul; you must stand before the emperor; and indeed, God has granted safety to all those who are sailing with you." So keep up your courage, men, for I have faith in God that it will be exactly as I have been told.
>
> (Acts 27:22–25)

Visions also have a broader, transformational agenda, motivating the recipients to align their lives with God's purposes.[38] As Ian Paul summarises, "Prophecy is less concerned with predicting the future in any abstract sense than with communicating God's message and calling people to obedience, by highlighting the consequences of their actions and the new possibilities offered by repentance and obedience."[39] A passage in Job (33:14–18) expresses this transformational intention very clearly:

> For God speaks in one way,
>   and in two, though people do not perceive it.

---

38 See e.g. Holmes, "Revelation," 773.
39 Paul, *Revelation*, 30.

> In a dream, in a vision of the night . . .
> . . . he opens their ears,
>   and terrifies them with warnings,
> that he may turn them aside from their deeds,
>   and keep them from pride,
> to spare their souls from the Pit,
>   their lives from traversing the River.

Motivational imagery of the future

We find a special type of vision report in the Bible which functions, in effect, as guided imagery (as discussed already in Chapter 3), generating "secondary" visions in the audience. One of the most prominent examples of this type is the vision of the promised land that Moses received and then shared with the whole Israelite community:

> For the Lord your God is bringing you into a good land, a land with flowing streams, with springs and underground waters welling up in valleys and hills, a land of wheat and barley, of vines and fig trees and pomegranates, a land of olive trees and honey, a land where you may eat bread without scarcity, where you will lack nothing, a land whose stones are iron and from whose hills you may mine copper. You shall eat your fill and bless the Lord your God for the good land that he has given you.
>
> (Deut 8:7–10)

Such guided imagery scripts have a salient motivational agenda; as shown in Chapter 2, imagined ideal future scenarios can exert considerable pulling power and can give the beholders hope; in this specific case the motivational purpose of Moses's script is also reflected by the warnings that frame the image: they remind people to "keep the commandments of the LORD your God, by walking in his ways and by fearing him" (v. 6) and then reiterate this warning after the vision (v. 11).

In a similar vein, the vibrant apocalyptic images that we find in several places in the Scriptures are not merely poetic descriptions for their own sake but also have an important motivational function. Some of the passages paint *utopian* pictures of an idyllic, peaceful and inclusive existence (e.g. Isaiah's visions of the renewal of the created order: 2:2–4; 11:6–9; 35:1–10; 65:17–25), thereby serving as desirable incentives. However, we have also seen in Chapter 2 that the emotional loading of *adverse* situations – that is, situations one would wish to avoid – can also be instrumental, as any hoped-for outcome will have a stronger motivational impact if the person is also reminded of the negative side of the coin, that is, what could happen if the desired state was *not* realised. This may explain why we also find in the Bible oracles portraying ruin and devastation (e.g. Zeph 1:14–18), stories like Lazarus and the Rich Man highlighting the torment in Hades (Luke 16:23), and images of judgment in the "hell of fire" (Matt 5:22)[40] that are associated with the "feared self": all these negative reminders can effectively complement the motivational potency of positive prospects. Indeed, even Moses's vision of the promised land (cited earlier) is juxtaposed with a warning that the Israelites should not forget God, "who brought you out of the land of Egypt, out of the house of slavery, who led you through the great and terrible wilderness, an arid wasteland with poisonous snakes and scorpions" (Deut 8:14–15). This warning acts as contrast and a reminder of the adverse alternative, and in order to ensure that there is no misunderstanding about the motivational intention of the passage, it concludes with this explicit admonition:

> If you do forget the Lord your God and follow other gods to serve and worship them, I solemnly warn you today that you shall surely perish. Like the nations that the Lord is destroying before you, so shall you perish, because you would not obey the voice of the Lord your God.
>
> (vv. 19–20)

The motivational character of prophetic imagination

We have briefly considered earlier Walter Brueggemann's proposal about prophetic imagination, according to which prophets engage in "futuring fantasy,"[41] that is, in creating an alternative world of possibilities. Brueggemann proposes that the prophet's vocation is to conjure up a reality that is "genuinely new and not derived,"[42] that is, to "construe, picture, and image reality outside of the dominant portrayals of reality."[43] This in turn helps to energise people and communities "by its promise of another time and situation toward which the community of faith may move."[44] This proposal is fully consistent with the motivational considerations outlined earlier, and so is Brueggemann's assertion that before prophets speak about possible futures that are to inspire the audience, they also picture the suffering and hurt that are present in the community or the disaster that is looming on the horizon.[45] Prophets thereby, in effect, "rock the boat" (see Chapter 2). In

---

40 The Greek word for "hell" here and in several other places is *geenna*, which is derived from the Hebrew place-name meaning "valley of Hinnom," a valley south of Jerusalem that was the place of child sacrifice to foreign gods. It was later used for dumping refuse, dead bodies of animals and executed criminals, with ongoing fires to consume the refuse. Thus, when a reference was made to "hell, where their worm never dies, and the fire is never quenched" (Mark 9:47–48), this would evoke a powerful image in Jewish audiences.
41 Brueggemann, *Prophetic Imagination*, 40.
42 Ibid., 14.
43 Brueggemann, *Theology of the Old Testament*, 625.
44 Brueggemann, *Prophetic Imagination*, 3.
45 Brueggemann, *Theology of the Old Testament*, 625–627.

this sense, prophetic practice closely reflects the complementary functions of positive and negative imagery of motivational vision, and this core combination of judgement and hope underlying prophetic messages is clearly expressed in Willem VanGemeren's summary:

> The prophets bore a *message of transformation* in a historical context to people who were complacent with their abilities and achievements. They spoke of God's imminent judgement on all humanity, including Israel and Judah, because humankind rebelled against the Lord, the King of Glory. They announced the *coming kingdom of the Lord*, the Judgement, and the *transformation of creation*. The *prophetic vision of God's glorious kingdom* shattered the reality of human kingdoms and structures but also shaped the vision of a remnant that lives in harmony with God.[46] (emphases added)

Summary

This chapter has presented biblical vision as one of the primary communication channels between the heavenly and the earthly spheres, one that humans can tune into in order to catch glimpses of some transcendent reality and to receive celestial messages. These celestial messages in the biblical corpus predominantly originate from, or are authorised by, God, as summarised in an oracle on divine communication reported in Numbers 12:6–8, where God declares that his means of communication with humans will involve the channel of vision as mediated by prophets.

The Scriptures highlight the involvement of the Holy Spirit in the perception of divine messages, and there is a prominent theological tradition going back to Origen and Augustine that connects the spirit-filled faculty of internal senses to the existence of an "inner man" in believers that orients them towards a growing likeness to God. Consistent with this conception, it was argued in the current chapter that equipping humans with the faculty of vision may be seen as core to God's act of making humankind in his image, thereby establishing an interface between the Creator and the creature.

We may gain further insight into the essence of biblical vision when we consider how the original circle of partakers in divine communication was widened in the biblical story. A prophecy to this effect presented in Joel 2:28–3:8 is declared by the Apostle Peter to have been fulfilled at Pentecost, enabling every disciple of Jesus to perceive communication from God directly. The numerous visionary experiences recorded in the New Testament bear abundant witness to the vital role played by the perception of vision in the advancement of Christianity.

---

46 VanGemeren, *Prophetic Word*, 19.

Finally, although references to vision are frequent in the Bible and visionary experiences occur in various forms, the specific purpose of most of these biblical visions is motivational in one way or another. The divine messages from God are authoritative as they are a manifestation of his will,[47] and vision reports that are conducive to "secondary" visualisation (i.e. evoke a visual experience in the audience) also have an abiding appeal.[48] Accordingly, James Packer's summary of divine revelation offers a fitting summary of the essence of vision:

> From the standpoint of its contents, divine revelation is both indicative and imperative, and in each respect normative. God's disclosures are always made in the context of a demand for trust in, and obedience to, what is revealed – a response, that is, which is wholly determined and controlled by the contents of the revelation itself. In other words, God's revelation comes to man, not as information without obligation, but as a mandatory rule of faith and conduct.[49]

Thus, the central feature of divine vision is to motivate people to respond to God's call and to guide them in the transformation process of being conformed to the image of Jesus (Rom 8:29).

References

Arnold, William T. 1996. "Visions." In *Evangelical Dictionary of Biblical Theology*, edited by Walter A. Elwell, 802–03. Grand Rapids, MI: Baker Books.

Augustine of Hippo. 2002. *On the Literal Meaning of Genesis* (in: *On Genesis*). Translated by Edmund Hill. New York: New City Press, 415.

Avis, Paul. 1999. *God and the Creative Imagination: Metaphor, Symbol and Myth in Religion and Theology*. London: Routledge.

Baker, David W. 2006. *Joel, Obadiah, Malachi*. NIV Application Commentary. Grand Rapids, MI: Zondervan.

Balthasar, Hans Urs von, ed. 1984. *Origen – Spirit and Fire: A Thematic Anthology of His Writings*. Edinburgh: T & T Clark.

Bock, Darrell L. 2007. *Acts*. Grand Rapids, MI: Baker Academic.

Boyd, Gregory A. 2004. *Seeing Is Believing: Experience Jesus through Imaginative Prayer*. Grand Rapids, MI: Baker Books.

Brueggemann, Walter. 1997. *Theology of the Old Testament: Testimony, Dispute, Advocacy*. Minneapolis, MN: Fortress.

Brueggemann, Walter. 2001. *The Prophetic Imagination*. 2nd ed. Minneapolis, MN: Fortress.

Carpenter, Eugene E., and Philip Wesley Comfort. 2000. *Holman Treasury of Key Bible Words: 200 Greek and 200 Hebrew Words Defined and Explained*. Nashville, TN: Broadman & Holman.

47 Carpenter and Comfort, *Key Bible Words*, 49.
48 Myers, "Vision," 1040–1041.
49 Packer, "Revelation," 1014.

Dailey, Patricia. 2012. "The Body and Its Senses." In *The Cambridge Companion to Christian Mysticism*, edited by Amy Hollywood and Patricia Zoltán Beckman, 264–76. Cambridge: Cambridge University Press.

deSilva, David A. 1997. "Visions, Ecstatic Experience." In *Dictionary of the Later New Testament and Its Developments*, edited by Ralph P. Martin and Peter H. Davids, 1194–98. Downers Grove, IL: InterVarsity Press.

Dörnyei, Zoltán, and Ema Ushioda. 2011. *Teaching and Researching Motivation*. 2nd ed. Harlow: Longman.

Dozeman, Thomas B. 1998. "The Book of Numbers: Introduction, Commentary and Reflections." In *The New Interpreter's Bible*, edited by Leander E. Keck, 1–268. Nashville, TN.

Everts, Janet Meyer. 1992. "Dreams in the New Testament and Greco-Roman Literature." In *The Anchor Bible Dictionary*, edited by David Noel Freedman, 231–31. New York: Doubleday.

Fraeters, Veerle. 2012. "Visio/Vision." In *The Cambridge Companion to Christian Mysticism*, edited by Amy Hollywood and Patricia Zoltán Beckman, 178–88. Cambridge: Cambridge University Press.

Guthrie, George H. 2015. *2 Corinthians*. Grand Rapids, MI: Baker Academic.

Harrison, Carol. 1999. "Senses, Spiritual." In *Augustine through the Ages: An Encyclopedia*, edited by Allan D. Fitzgerald, 767–68. Grand Rapids, MI: Eerdmans.

Holmes, Stephen R. 2016. "Revelation." In *New Dictionary of Theology: Historic and Systematic*, edited by Martin Davie, Tim Grass, Stephen R. Holmes, John McDowell and T. A. Noble, 770–73. Downers Grove, IL: IVP Academic.

Hubbard, David A. 1989. *Joel and Amos: An Introduction and Commentary*. Tyndale Old Testament Commentaries 25. Downers Grove, IL: IVP Academic.

Humphrey, Edith M. 2007. *And I Turned to See the Voice: The Rhetoric of Vision in the New Testament*. Grand Rapids, MI: Baker Academic.

Marshall, I. Howard. 1980. *Acts: An Introduction and Commentary*. Nottingham: Inter-Varsity Press.

Miller, John B. F. 2013. "Dreams and Visions." In *Dictionary of Jesus and the Gospels; Second Edition* edited by Joel B. Green, Jeannine K. Brown and Norman Perrin, 216–18. Downers Grove, IL: IVP Academic.

Myers, Allen C. 1987. "Vision." In *The Eerdmans Bible Dictionary*, edited by Allen C. Myers, 1040–41. Grand Rapids, MI: Eerdmans.

Packer, J. I. "Revelation." In *New Bible Dictionary*, edited by I. Howard Marshall, A. R. Millard, J. I. Packer and D. J. Wiseman. 1014–16. Downers Grove, IL: InterVarsity Press, 1996.

Paul, Ian. 2018. *Revelation*. London: Inter-Varsity Press.

Rahner, Karl. 1963. *Visions and Prophecies*. Translated by Charles H. Henkey and Richard Strachan. Freiburg: Herder.

Stuart, Charles, M. 1915. "Vision." In *The International Standard Bible Encyclopaedia*, edited by J. Orr, J. L. Nuelsen, E. Y. Mullins and M. O. Evans, 3057–58. Chicago: The Howard-Severance Company.

Stuart, Douglas. 1987. *Hosea – Jonah*. Word Biblical Commentary 31. Dallas: Word.

VanGemeren, Willem. 1990. *Interpreting the Prophetic Word: An Introduction to the Prophetic Literature of the Old Testament*. Grand Rapids, MI: Zondervan.

Wenham, Gordon J. 1981. *Numbers: An Introduction and Commentary*. Tyndale Old Testament Commentaries 4. Downers Grove, IL: IVP Academic.

Wright, Robert E. 1999. "Mysticism." In *Augustine through the Ages: An Encyclopedia*, edited by Allan D. Fitzgerald, 576–80. Grand Rapids, MI: Eerdmans.

5   The vulnerability and authentication of divine vision

The overview of biblical vision in the previous chapters has shown that visionary experiences occur frequently and in many forms in the Bible, and that they also include prophetic practices in general. We have seen that the divine messages delivered through the channel of vision are often depicted in the Scriptures as playing a decisive role in shaping the history of humanity. This significance was aptly reflected at one of the key events of the emergence of the Christian faith, Pentecost: when the Apostle Peter gave a speech to the bewildered crowd to explain the happenings, he began by highlighting vision as an integral part of the powerful intervention of God, inextricably linked to the release of the Holy Spirit amongst the disciples of Jesus. At the same time, the centrality of prophetic vision in Christianity has also been in direct correlation with the gravity of the damage that false prophecy could potentially cause, and the biblical corpus contains multiple warnings about the fact that divine messages might be misconceived or falsely claimed. A good illustration of this twofold situation is offered by the Apostle Paul's disposition: while he actively encouraged believers to strive for the spiritual gift of prophesy (1 Cor 14:1) and thus to become, in effect, visionaries themselves, he also repeatedly underlined the need to test every prophecy carefully (1 Thess 5:20–21; 1 Cor 14:29). That this was not an empty warning is evidenced by the fact that, as Newman recounts, even some of the most venerated recipients of divine vision in the past "lived in dread of delusion;"[1] for example, the medieval Franciscan mystic Angela of Foligno (1248–1309), who became known as "Mistress of Theologians" and who has been canonised by the Catholic church, was convinced from time to time that she was possessed by demons, and Newman also reports that the renowned English mystic, Julian of Norwich (1342–1416), had initially doubted her own spontaneous visions, "believing that she had 'raved' in the grip of a life-threatening illness."[2] Accordingly, we shall start this chapter by taking a closer look at the possible vulnerabilities and limitations

---

1 Newman, "Medieval Visionary Culture," 35.
2 Ibid.

of vision, and then follow with an overview of the procedures established in the Bible as well as in church tradition for the purpose of authenticating divine visionary content.

The vulnerability of vision

Chapter 3 concluded about divine vision reports that they always contain a human element, which is consistent with the Apostle Paul's assertion that "we know only in part, and we prophesy only in part" (1 Cor 13:9). It was argued that although this does not necessarily render the reports inaccurate, it does constitute a potential vulnerability, because the human contribution may distort the divine content and, more importantly, the distortion may also be affected by spiritual interference from forces pursuing agendas contrary to God's. In this section we shall examine these two sources of vulnerability and then discuss whether we can take the bodily signs of a religious experience that accompany the reception of a vision as an indication of the authenticity of the message.

Subjective distortion

Jeremiah 23:16 makes a harsh denunciation of false prophets: "Thus says the Lord of hosts: Do not listen to the words of the prophets who prophesy to you; they are deluding you. They speak visions of their own minds." The noteworthy aspect of this condemnation for the current discussion is that it does not accuse false prophets of "lying" or "making things up" (as would be the case, for example, with false witnesses in a court case) but rather of "speaking visions of their own minds"; in a similar vein, Ezekiel 13:2–3 also speaks about false prophets "who prophesy out of their own imagination . . . who follow their own spirit." In other words, false prophets may report visions they genuinely experience, but these visions are internally generated rather than externally provided by God. As we saw in Chapter 1, science locates the ultimate source of mental imagery in the visionary's own subconscious, a point underlined by Boyd very clearly: "The fundamental assumption behind modern science and most modern psychology is that everything that takes place in your mind is all your doing. . . . The only pictures we can receive are the ones we create."[3] Moreover, it is also established in science that humans can deliberately conjure up visions by directing their minds to engage in visualisation, and thus vision in science is conceived of as a sometimes self-induced mental creation that utilises subconscious/ implicit memories and knowledge. The earlier quotations from Jeremiah and Ezekiel suggest that this is exactly how some false prophets operated

3 Boyd, *Seeing Is Believing*, 196.

and then convinced themselves that their imagined picture or scenario was of divine origin.[4]

These considerations corroborate the suggestion made by William McKane (amongst others) that in at least some cases false prophets did not perpetrate a deliberate fraud: "They are not guilty of a calculated deceit, but they are deluded, for they equate the vividness and strength of their own insights and visions with the word of Yahweh."[5] Martin Buber succinctly summarises these cases by stating that "the false prophets make their subconscious a god, whereas for the true prophets their subconscious is subdued by the God of truth."[6] The matter, however, is not entirely black and white, because even with the best of intentions there may not exist a 100% "true" vision: as we have seen when discussing vision reports in Chapter 3, when a vision is perceived, interpreted and then verbalised by a human recipient, the outcome will inevitably contain some degree of subjective personal element. Walter Kaiser offers a pertinent biblical illustration of this point:[7] in 2 Samuel 7:3 the prophet Nathan – who is presented in the Bible as a true prophet – tells David that he can go ahead and build the temple, "for the Lord is with you." However, the same night Nathan receives God's word that he has miscommunicated God's will, because it is David's son who will build God's house (v. 13), a message which Nathan duly conveys to David (v. 17).

Accordingly, many theologians throughout the centuries have shared Rahner's conclusion that the content of divine vision "will inevitably represent the joint effect of the divine influence plus all the subjective dispositions of the visionary."[8] Rahner lists convincing examples which show that even established vision reports whose authenticity has been ascertained by ecclesiastic authorities might contain not only subjective but also "erroneous and bizarre" elements.[9] Indeed, Benedict Groeschel points out that

---

4 Another relevant biblical passage that allows this reading is Lam 2:14: "Your prophets have seen for you false and deceptive visions; they have . . . seen oracles for you that are false and misleading."

5 McKane, *Jeremiah*, 578–579.

6 Buber, *Prophetic Faith*, 179; he further argues that although false prophets are sometimes motivated to please the people who inquire on them, at other times they wish to please their own "dream" and "phantom"; that is, "they do not simply deceive on purpose, but they themselves are entangled in the delusion of the world of wish."

7 Kaiser, "False Prophets," 243.

8 Rahner, *Visions and Prophecies*, 63; see also Groeschel, *Reported Revelations*, 95. Likewise, Proudfoot's (*Religious Experience*, 228) conclusion about religious experience in general also applies to visions: "Religious experience cannot be identified without reference to concepts, beliefs, grammatical rules, and practices." As he elaborates, "What must be explained is why they understood what happened to them or what they witnessed in religious terms. This requires a mapping of the concepts and beliefs that were available to them, the commitments they brought to the experience, and the contextual conditions that might have supported their identification of their experiences in religious terms" (p. 226).

9 Rahner, *Visions and Prophecies*, 72.

there has been a clear papal teaching for centuries that "even a canonized saint who has reported a private revelation which has been approved by the Church . . . may have introduced some personal element that is subject to error or distortion."[10] Rahner further emphasises in this respect that the distortive intrusion of subjective content may not necessarily occur at the perception stage but may also happen *after* the visionary experience:

> even in the case of perfectly honest people: unconscious corrections, tricks of memory, the use of pre-established mental patterns and a familiar vocabulary in the account which will imperceptibly shift the perspective, unconscious later additions, psychological description and interpretation of the event which will be more or less successful according to the seer's capacity for self-analysis.[11]

Divination and diabolical influence

Jeremiah 14:14 presents the same message as in 23:16 (cited earlier), but with one important addition: here "divination" is also added to the false prophets' actions:

> And the Lord said to me: The prophets are prophesying lies in my name; I did not send them, nor did I command them or speak to them. They are prophesying to you a lying vision, worthless divination, and the deceit of their own minds.

The Hebrew term translated as "divination" (*qě'·sěm*) can be defined as "the pagan state or process of stating or determining the future (or hidden knowledge) through signs, omens, and supernatural powers."[12] The attitude of the Bible towards divination is consistently negative, strictly forbidding it[13] – Deuteronomy 18:10–14 expresses this prohibition in no uncertain terms and describes the practice of divination alongside other forms of magic and witchcraft as "abhorrent to the Lord," concluding: "You must remain completely loyal to the Lord your God. Although these nations that you are about to dispossess do give heed to soothsayers and diviners, as for you, the Lord your God does not permit you to do so" (vv. 13–14). We should note that this passage does *not* deny the existence or

---

10 Groeschel, *Reported Revelations*, 27.
11 Rahner, *Visions and Prophecies*, 75. Hamon (*Dreams and Visions*, 59) argues in a similar vein: "many well-meaning Christians have been led astray in their personal lives by incorrectly interpreting revelation given to them through dreams, visions, prophecies or even by a still, small inner voice, which they believe to be God's voice but, rather, might be their own unhealed, deceitful hearts speaking to them."
12 Swanson, *Dictionary of Biblical Languages*.
13 See e.g. Van Dam, "Divination," 162.

the power of divination but only declares that God's people should refrain from receiving any spiritual message that is not of divine origin. This prohibition thus indirectly confirms that there are spiritual forces that are not following God's divine purpose and which are capable of interfering with the human faculty of mental imagery. We are indeed warned in Scripture not only that Satan is "the deceiver of the whole world" (Rev 12:9) but that he may disguise himself as an angel of light (1 Cor 11:14), and one way of doing so may involve delivering fake messages disguised as divine. In fact, Jesus himself forewarned the disciples that "many false prophets will arise and lead many astray" (Matt 24:11).

In the Middle Ages visionary experiences took on an increasingly prominent role in church life, as a result of which there was a proliferation of instances of mystical ecstasies producing reports of highly questionable "divine" encounters.[14] In order to develop a solid theological foundation for the purpose of discerning any possible diabolical deception behind these visions, the church went back to Augustine's extensive work on vision for advice, particularly to *On the Literal Meaning of Genesis*.[15] In this book, Augustine took a cautious stance as he believed it was possible that "evil ones deceive by means both of bodily vision and of the images of bodily realities which are exhibited in the spirit."[16] The great visionary Ignatius of Loyola (to be discussed in the next chapter) also reported in his *Autobiography* a frequent "beautiful" appearance in his visions that he later identified as the devil, which had to be consciously dispelled.[17] All this created a general disposition in the church towards visionary imagination that was bordering between wariness and outright suspicion,[18] and this climate surrounding vision has prevailed in church practice to date. In a contemporary guide to revelations, for example, Groeschel stresses that "great caution

---

14 Elliott, "Raptus/Rapture," 197.

15 Augustine (*On the Literal Meaning of Genesis*, 464–506) devotes the whole of the final book of this work (Book XII) to a discussion of vision, triggered by Paul's journey to Paradise in the third heaven (2 Cor 12:2–4). For a summary of the church's turn to Augustine, see Fraeters, "Vision/Vision," 188; Newman, "Medieval Visionary Culture," 6.

16 Augustine, *On the Literal Meaning of Genesis*, 12.29 (p. 479).

17 Ignatius, *Autobiography*, cited in McGinn, *Christian Mysticism*, 356: "While kneeling before a nearby cross to give thanks to God, there appeared to him [i.e. to Ignatius] that object he had often seen before, but had never understood. It seemed to be something most beautiful, and, as it were, gleaming with many eyes. This is how it always appeared. While before the cross, he clearly noticed that the object did not have its former beautiful colour. He understood clearly with strong agreement of his will that it was the devil. Later, whenever the vision appeared to him for a long time, as it did often, with contempt he dispelled it with the staff he used to carry in his hand." (The *Autobiography* is the transcription of Ignatius's spoken narrative in the third person by Father Gonzales.)

18 A telling illustration of this point is Elliott's ("Raptus/Rapture," 197) report that Bonaventure, who became master general of the Franciscan order, remained hostile to visions, believing them to be "more to be feared than desired," despite the fact that "Francis's stigmata were administered by a seraph during the course of an ecstasy."

must be exercised with reports of visions because self-delusion or even dia-bolical influence is apparently common in such things."[19]

Religious experience and the validation of vision

The discussion of *religious experience* in relation to the vulnerability of vision is warranted by its potential to cover up distortion or deception in the sense that such experiences may be considered hallmarks of genuine heavenly vision. As has already been mentioned, visionary experiences are sometimes accompanied by various forms of altered states of consciousness (e.g. trances), and starting in the Middle Ages, Christian visionaries increasingly relied on conscious inducement techniques of enhanced religious experiences, because they regarded these as gateways to receiving divine vision. In describing the emerging trend, Newman explains that from the 12th century onwards, visionary experience was "not a spontaneous, wholly unpredictable incursion of the divine into the world." Rather, she continues, "it was a privileged cultural practice by which those with appro-priate qualifications – at first only monks and nuns, later beguines and ter-tiaries, eventually even devout laypeople – might court sacred encounters through techniques for the deliberate alteration of consciousness."[20]

This practice made waves and generated considerable controversy in the Middle Ages, yet the phenomenon of inducing enhanced personal states that facilitate mental imagery was not new – Chapter 1, for example, reviewed Erika Bourguignon's anthropological survey that showed the widespread use of consciously generated visionary experiences in most known histori-cal cultures. Although the Bible is reticent about such ecstatic practices,[21] we find some allusions to a link between vision and prophetic ecstasy in the fact that the Hebrew verb "to prophesy" (*nābā'*) is associated in a few places with ecstatic behaviour rather than merely receiving or conveying God's message[22] (e.g. Num 11:25[23]), so much so that the NRSV, for exam-ple, sometimes translates the verb as "to rave" (e.g. 1 Kgs 18:29) or "to be in a prophetic frenzy" (e.g. 1 Sam 10:5, 10; 19:20–21, 22–24). In a similar vein, Jeremiah 29:26 likens a prophet to a madman: ". . . so that there may be officers in the house of the Lord to control any madman who plays the prophet." In his overview of biblical ecstasy, Aune offers a further point to support the existence of a distinct ecstatic state associated with proph-ets, namely that the onset of this revelatory state tends to be marked by

19 Groeschel, *Reported Revelations*, 150.
20 Newman, "Medieval Visionary Culture," 5–6.
21 See e.g. Hultgård, "Ecstasy and Vision," 220; in fact, Dunn ("Biblical Concepts of Revela-tion," 11) argues that "there seems to have been some reaction against the potential abuse of prophecy so conceived."
22 See e.g. Ashley, *Book of Numbers*, 213–214.
23 The Greek word for "to prophesy" (*prophēteuō*) is used in a similar meaning in Acts 19:6.

"stereotyped" phrases such as "the Spirit of God came upon" someone or "the hand of the Lord came/was upon" someone, thereby distinguishing these conditions from the normal state of consciousness.[24]

Thus, there is an unquestionable association between religious experience and the perception of vision, but as was argued when reviewing this matter from a scientific perspective in Chapter 1, this relationship is based only on the frequent co-occurrence of the two phenomena rather than on a causative link: because bodily senses dim the operation of mental imagery, switching off physical sensation by a trance can create an optimal neuroscientific condition for perceiving a vision.[25] It shows the clarity of Augustine's thinking on the subject that he stated over 1500 years ago that ecstasy can help to focus on the spiritual or intellectual vision.[26] This association, however, does not mean that an altered state of consciousness is a prerequisite to any visionary experience, let alone a guarantee of the authenticity of a divine vision. And yet, it appears that signs of religious experience have been taken throughout the centuries as a mark of the validity of the divine spiritual content of a vision. We should recall that false prophets in Old Testament times were sometimes deluded by the vividness and strength of their own imagery into thinking that those were of divine origin, and as David Seal explains, the false prophets' self-induced ecstatic state was perceived by many "as seizure by the Spirit of God."[27] Accordingly, as Seal sums up, "Viewers would thus interpret whatever utterances the false prophets made while in this state as expressions of God's will."[28] A notable biblical example of the close association between prophetic frenzy and being regarded as a genuine prophet is offered in 1 Samuel 19:23–24:

> and the spirit of God came upon him [Saul]. As he was going, he fell into a prophetic frenzy, until he came to Naioth in Ramah. He too stripped off his clothes, and he too fell into a frenzy before Samuel. He lay naked all that day and all that night. Therefore it is said, "Is Saul also among the prophets?"
>
> (1 Sam 19:23–24)

---

24 Aune, "Ecstasy," 15.
25 This point is clearly summed up by Colleen Shantz (*Paul in Ecstasy*, 115): "In the normal brain, ecstatic visions are . . . made possible when their door is shut against the external world. Trance states are one way to shut that door."
26 Augustine, *On the Literal Meaning of Genesis*, 12.25 (p. 477): "When, however, the attention of the mind is totally turned aside and snatched away from the senses of the body, then you have what is more usually called ecstasy. Then whatever bodies may be there in front of the subject, even with his eyes wide open he simply does not see them at all, or of course hear any words spoken aloud. His attention is wholly taken up in gazing either at the images of bodies with the spiritual kind of vision, or with the intellectual kind at incorporeal realities that no bodily image can represent."
27 Seal, "Prophetic Ecstasy."
28 Ibid.

This passage shows that even as unlikely a candidate as King Saul was considered by some to be a prophet (though incredulously) on account of the bodily manifestations he displayed during his trance. A similar link between religious experience and divine vision also prevailed in the Middle Ages, as is illustrated by Newman's summary of medieval monastery practices:

> The visionary subculture par excellence was the monastery, where constant immersion in Scripture, exegesis, hagiography, and contemplative writings trained the monk or nun to accept the possibility, or even likelihood, of visions and to esteem them highly. Visionary experience was never supposed to be an end in itself, at least not in principle: it was valued because it could lead the soul into deeper contrition, purer devotion, more perfect knowledge, and greater intimacy with God. Nevertheless, visions and ecstasies were always treated in hagiography as signs of divine favour, and competition for these graces could be intense.[29]

It appears therefore that ecstatic states have been widely seen as signs of "divine favour" over the centuries, despite the fact that, as seen in Chapter 1, some degree of altered states of consciousness can be relatively easily induced with some practice. This is thus an area undoubtedly open to potential abuse, and as Luke Timothy Johnson alerts us, there have indeed been many cases in church history when people faked religious experiences for one reason or another.[30] This gives extra weight to Jesus' warning in Mark 13:22: "False messiahs and false prophets will appear and produce signs and omens, to lead astray, if possible, the elect."

The other side of the coin

Despite the fact that the content of vision is vulnerable to distortion and deception, and that visionary experiences are not safe against abuse, Rahner, along with many other theologians, emphasises that vision must not be sidelined, as it forms an integral part of the Christian faith.[31] Indeed, without keeping the channel of divine communication open, Christian believers would not be able to benefit from the teaching of the Holy Spirit that Jesus promised and which is to be delivered, presumably at least in part, through the visionary channel: "But the Advocate, the Holy Spirit, whom the Father will send in my name, will teach you everything, and remind you of all that I have said to you" (John 14:26). Jesus later elaborated on this as follows:

> I still have many things to say to you, but you cannot bear them now. When the Spirit of truth comes, he will guide you into all the truth; for

29 Newman, "Medieval Visionary Culture," 14.
30 Johnson, *Religious Experience*, 53.
31 Rahner, *Visions and Prophecies*, 15.

he will not speak on his own, but will speak whatever he hears, and he will declare to you the things that are to come. He will glorify me, because he will take what is mine and declare it to you.

(John 16:12–14)

It is also appropriate to reiterate here Moses's wish "that all the Lord's people were prophets, and that the Lord would put his spirit on them!" (Num 11:29) as well as Paul's teaching that believers should "Pursue love and strive for the spiritual gifts, and especially that you may prophesy" (1 Cor 14:1). In fact, Ephesians 2:19–20 declares that the "household of God [is] built upon the foundation of the apostles and prophets." Thus, given that humans are hard-wired to experience mental imagery and that aspects of this faculty are part of our basic cognitive operations such as memory functions, the question as to whether we should or should not practice mental imagery may simply be misplaced. Rather, the real issue is *how* we can ensure that the human faculty of vision is used to good effect and that it is not hijacked by personal subjectivity, wishful thinking or powers that represent agendas other than God's. Rahner articulates this dilemma very clearly:

An experience alleged to be a vision simply cannot compel one either to accept it as accurate in every detail, or to reject it altogether as a human or diabolical illusion or fraud. Such a logical and plausible rigorism is in fact a psychological blunder. From our point of view a certain leniency and a disposition to grant the divine origin of visionary experiences even if their whole content cannot be admitted, is quite defensible. It is not absolutely impossible, indeed, that pure hallucination and genuine visions might occur in the same person.[32]

The same dilemma underlies Paul's twofold warning in 1 Thess 5:19–21 that on the one hand, believers should not "quench the Spirit" and "despise the words of prophets," but on the other hand, they should "test every-thing." Moreover, Boyd rightly reminds us in this respect that although the biblical authors consistently spoke about the dangers of false prophecy, we do not find a single recommendation in the Scriptures that we should ban or avoid prophecy in general.[33] His conclusion about this conflicting issue offers a measured stance:

Given Satan's persuasive influence in the world, the existence of coun-terfeits should not surprise us. . . . The presence of false visions no more disqualifies the existence of true visions than does the presence of false messiahs disqualify the existence of a true Messiah. When we think in

32 Ibid., 74.
33 Boyd, *Seeing Is Believing*, 133.

this way and "throw the baby out with the bath water," we are simply giving in to the tactic of the enemy. To be sure, Christians need to be careful to stand firmly on the truth and to guard against error. Yet they need to be equally careful that they do not overreact in the retreat from error to the point that they also compromise the truth![34]

Authenticating divine vision

The previous discussion explains why the authentication of divine vision has been an acute issue for the church over the centuries; indeed, David Lonsdale rightly states that "discernment lies at the heart of Christian spirituality."[35] Because of the explicit biblical ban on various forms of divination and witchcraft, it is relatively straightforward to exclude from the range of legitimate visionary practices all the illicit means of discerning "otherworldly" information, such as, for example, King Saul's asking the witch of Endor to "bring up" the dead Samuel so that he could inquire of him what to do (1 Sam 28:7–12). However, the validation task is much harder with vision reports that come from respectable sources and which present content that does not flag up immediate issues. In such cases, the discernment of any possible human contribution, and especially potential errors and deception, requires subtle procedures, and we find several possible testing methods both in the Scriptures and in church practice for this purpose. We should note here, though, that none of these procedures are entirely foolproof, which is also reflected in the subtitle of the Catholic church's protocol for the ecclesiastical approbation of divine vision: "Criteria for judging, *at least with probability*, the character of the presumed apparitions or revelations"[36] (emphasis added).

The following discussion of possible authentication procedures will be centred around four aspects of the visionary experience: the vision's (a) *recipient*, (b) *content* and (c) *consequences*, as well as (d) methods of *external verification*. In order to illustrate the authentication process and its limitations, the chapter will conclude with an extended validity check of one rather ambiguous vision report in the Bible, Eliphaz's nocturnal visitation in the Book of Job (4:12–21), applying the various criteria of authenticity considered before.[37]

The recipient of the vision

In opposing false prophets, Jeremiah declares that only those who had stood in the council of the Lord are true prophets (Jer 23:18, 22), and one such

---

34 Ibid.
35 Lonsdale, *Eyes to See*, 89.
36 Sacred Congregation for the Doctrine of the Faith, *Norms Regarding Discernment*.
37 For a more detailed version of this analysis, see Chapter 5 in Dörnyei, *Progressive Creation*, 140–151; 164–169.

visionary experience – by the prophet Micaiah – is described in the Old Testament (1 Kgs 22:19–23). It would seem however, that this criterion for the authenticity of vision applies only to the pre-Pentecostal period, when the faculty of receiving divine communication was activated only for a select group of prophets. A more pertinent test for the current era regarding the recipient of the vision is to examine the personal qualities of the visionary, most importantly his/her mental condition, personal integrity and spiritual standing. According to the guidelines of the Catholic church, the required individual characteristics in this respect include "psychological equilibrium, honesty and rectitude of moral life, sincerity and habitual docility towards Ecclesiastical Authority."[38] Consequently, Rahner concludes that the vision of someone who is well-balanced, theologically trained and "uninterested in certain dangerous subjects (divination)" is likely to be viewed as more reliable, even though he admits that it does not guarantee a greater divine influence in their case than in the case of others.[39]

As a further consideration, Rahner also cites the conviction of the renowned visionary St. Teresa of Ávila (1515–1582) that "if a person has once experienced a real vision he can never again be deceived by hallucinations,"[40] thereby underlining the issue of the visionary's accumulated experience. Indeed, the familiarity with God's voice is a biblical concept, highlighted in Jesus' teaching about the sheep knowing and recognising the shepherd's voice in John's Gospel (10:3, 14, 27), where we specifically read: "they will never follow a stranger; in fact, they will run away from him because they do not recognize a stranger's voice" (v. 5). Hebrews 5:14 affirms that the human capability of distinguishing good from evil can be "trained by practice," and John 7:17 also suggests that a mature Christian will be able to tell if a message is fake: "Anyone who resolves to do the will of God will know whether the teaching is from God or whether I am speaking on my own." In Ignatian spirituality (to be discussed in the next chapter), a central concept of spiritual discernment is "*sentir*," referring to an intuitive "felt-knowledge" or resonance that one can develop with practice and which, in turn, will signal attunement with the Holy Spirit.[41] Yet, we should note that despite knowing Ignatius's teachings intimately, Rahner has still argued that not even seemingly genuine internal experiences can offer complete guarantee against error,[42] and this susceptibility is consistent with the fact reported earlier that even the accounts of canonised mystics have been subject to error and distortion.[43]

38 Sacred Congregation for the Doctrine of the Faith, *Norms Regarding Discernment.*
39 Rahner, *Visions and Prophecies*, 65.
40 Ibid.
41 See e.g. Futrell, "Ignatian Discernment," 56–57.
42 Rahner, *Visions and Prophecies*, 65.
43 Futrell ("Ignatian Discernment," 60) reminds us that even Ignatius, who undoubtedly had a highly developed understanding of mystical experiences, warned of the difficulty of

The Orthodox church has traditionally discouraged the use of any form of mental imagery and has been, by and large, opposed to sensory imagination during prayer altogether.[44] Yet, there have been some notable exceptions reported amongst the Orthodox saints, and in his analysis, Sergei Sveshnikov submits that in their cases what safeguarded the purity of their visions was their ongoing prayer of repentance and humility[45] (i.e. the coverage of the Jesus Prayer, "Lord Jesus Christ, Son of God, have mercy on me, a sinner"). In contrast, the western church tradition has displayed a less restrictive approach; it was already mentioned that, starting in the Middle Ages, there was a growing circle of devout believers who would consciously strive to engender visionary experiences, disregarding the potential corruption of visions and trusting the Lord to protect them from deception. Romans 8:26 is repeatedly cited as a justification of this belief – "the Spirit helps us in our weakness; for we do not know how to pray as we ought, but that very Spirit intercedes with sighs too deep for words"[46] – and Newman explains that visionaries who cultivated visionary experiences "envisaged an implicit synergy between grace and human effort, and, without altogether discounting the wiles of demons, . . . expressed confidence in the devotee's ability to expose and defeat them with the help of God."[47] An interesting twist of this approach is the adoption of an initially sceptical attitude as a default position, praying to God for priming only that part of the content of a vision that really originates from him and not from other sources; the influential Jesuit writer on prayer, Thomas Green, for example states the following:

> Thus I have found it quite safe, and pleasing to the Lord, to say to him: "Lord, if these thoughts and images are really from you, you insist on them. But since it is more likely that I am the source of them and they are interfering with your work in me, I will continue quietly to push them aside."[48]

The content of the vision

The Bible offers only limited guidance on how to validate the *content* of a vision. Deuteronomy 18:21 addresses the question of how to tell apart true and false prophecy: "You may say to yourself, 'How can we recognize

---

distinguishing between authentic divine visions and their consequent "'afterglow,' when one's own ideas and opinions, which are not immediately from God, come to the foreground of consciousness."

44 Sveshnikov, *Imagine That*, 26.
45 Ibid., 38.
46 E.g. Gallagher (*Meditation and Contemplation*, 38) states, "We trust, then, that the Spirit, who 'comes to the aid our weakness' (Rom. 8:26) when we pray, will guide not only the activity of our minds, but also the work of our imaginations."
47 Newman, "Medieval Visionary Culture," 6.
48 Green, *When the Well Runs Dry*, 150–151.

a word that the Lord has not spoken?' " The answer given is that what the prophet says must come to pass (v. 22), but this condition is further qualified in Deuteronomy 13:1–3, which states that even if a prophecy does take place, one must not heed the word of the prophet if he/she leads people to serve "other gods" (v. 2). Thus, the truthfulness of a prediction as a criterion – which, we should note, may be relevant only to some visions, and even then it is not always straightforward what timeframe to use for expecting the fulfilment – is cancelled if the prophet is not true to God and leads people away from him. This last point is related to the *fruit* of the vision, which will be addressed in the next section.

The paucity of direct biblical teaching about authentic vision content is offset, however, by the rich but indirect validation standards that are offered by the Bible itself. It probably does not require much justification that the primary criterion concerning the substance of an authentic divine vision is that it should be in harmony with previously revealed biblical truths; for example, the second main criterion set up by the Catholic church's protocol for judging the character of a vision is "true theological and spiritual doctrine and immune from error."[49] In order to put this criterion into context, let us reiterate briefly the biblical progression of safeguarding divine communication, as discussed in Chapter 4:

- God spoke to his most trusted servant, Moses, in plain words.
- During the period between Moses and Jesus' ministry, God communicated only to a select group of prophets, and even with them he used an enhanced mode of communication (applying vision or riddles) that increased the power of the divine messages.
- During Jesus' earthly ministry, God spoke only through his Son, who was "the image of the invisible God" (Col 1:15). This mode of communication was even more enhanced than relying on mental imagery, because it moved from *imagined* to *actual reality* – after all, "the Word became flesh" (John 1:14) and therefore the embodied channel of divine communication actually "lived among us, and we have seen his glory" (v. 14). Without wanting to be frivolous, the move changed the "audiovisual" quality of God's visionary messages into a "high definition" or "3D format," and it is also underlined in Acts 2:22 that Jesus was "attested to you [or "validated"[50]] by God with deeds of power, wonders, and signs." Accordingly, during this period God's communication could not have been any more secure.
- After Pentecost, the activation of the human faculty of vision in believers through the release of the indwelling Spirit resulted in a new security situation: the earlier protection of divine vision through the tight

---

49 Sacred Congregation for the Doctrine of the Faith, *Norms Regarding Discernment;* see also e.g. Kaiser, "False Prophets," 242.
50 Hart, *New Testament: A Translation,* 223.

control of who could become a visionary was replaced by a seemingly more relaxed criterion, namely that the recipient of divine communication had to be a *follower of Jesus*. This widening of the circle of visionaries increased the risk of any potential mishandling of vision and thus inevitably shifted the onus of protecting the authenticity of vision onto guarding its *content*.

How was it possible to start exercising a tighter control over visionary content when, as we saw earlier, the Jewish canon of Scripture did not provide detailed guidelines in this respect? The answer lies in two additional factors that are related specifically to New Testament times:

- First, we must remember that the Great Commission stipulated that in order to qualify to be a disciple of Jesus – that is, to become eligible to have access to vision – one had to learn "everything" that Jesus had taught to the initial Twelve (Matt 28:20).
- Second, the body of Christian knowledge signified by this stipulation became increasingly formalised within a generation after Pentecost with the emergence of the new Christian canon of Scripture, the New Testament.

Consequently, the New Testament could act as a detailed compendium of Christian knowledge against which the content of a vision could be evaluated. As such, it established a solid criterion for checking whether or not the content of a vision was in harmony with previously revealed biblical truths, and thus constituted, in effect, a firm new filter of protection.

The consequences of the vision

The third main point of the Catholic church's protocol for discernment specifies that a vision should lead to "spiritual fruit,"[51] thereby foregrounding the *consequences* of a vision. This is a subject that the New Testament addresses in several places, starting with the Sermon on the Mount, where Jesus specifically speaks about discernment between true and false prophets, warning people that truth can be violated:[52] "Beware of false prophets, who come to you in sheep's clothing but inwardly are ravenous wolves. You will know them *by their fruits*" (Matt 7:15–16; emphasis added).[53] This evaluation principle is reiterated for emphasis in v. 20: "Thus you will know them by their fruits." In other words, Jesus taught that the real value

51 Sacred Congregation for the Doctrine of the Faith, *Norms Regarding Discernment*: "Healthy devotion and abundant and constant spiritual fruit (for example, spirit of prayer, conversion, testimonies of charity, etc.)."
52 Carson, "Matthew," 227.
53 See also Jesus' teaching on "The Tree and Its Fruit" in Luke 6:43–45.

of something is reflected in what it leads to, and *mutatis mutandi*, a vision's value is reflected by the quality of impact it makes. This is a recurring theme in Jesus' teaching, and in Matthew 2:33–37 he also applied it to people in general: "The good person brings good things out of a good treasure, and the evil person brings evil things out of an evil treasure" (v. 35; see also Luke 6:45). In fact, the instruction in Deuteronomy 13:1–3 (cited earlier) that one must not listen to the words of prophets who lead people away from God is based on the same principle, namely that the measure of someone should be taken by the consequences of his/her deeds.

The Apostle Paul's declaration about prophecy in 1 Corinthians 14:3 – "those who prophesy speak to other people for their upbuilding and encouragement and consolation" – also concerns the desired impact of prophetic vision and it can thus help to further specify its purpose: authentic prophecy ought to have a beneficial and edifying impact that builds up the recipient. Rahner expounds on this important condition as follows:

> The good in every prophecy is ultimately shown if it awakens us to the gravity of decision in courageous faith, if it makes clear to us that the world is in a deplorable state (which we never like to admit), if it steels our patience and fortifies our faith that God has already triumphed, even if in this world we still have distress, if it fills us with confidence in the one Lord of the still secret future, if it brings us to prayer, to conversion of heart, and to faith that nothing shall separate us from the love of Christ.[54]

Methods of external verification

We saw in Chapter 4 that the most important visionary experiences of the Apostles Paul and Peter that played a vital role in the emergence of Christianity were accompanied by "paired visions," that is, by independent visions corroborating each other. This is a powerful form of verification, because each vision acts, in effect, as an external control for the other, which can help to eliminate any personal, subjective distortions or misunderstandings of the visionary message. It also makes it more unlikely – although does not completely rule out the possibility – that both messages have been affected by spiritual interference in a parallel manner.[55] Of course, such paired visions cannot be orchestrated directly by humans as a method of

---

54 Rahner, *Visions and Prophecies*, 106.
55 It is relevant in this respect that, as Hamon (*Dreams and Visions*, 68) highlights, repeated or similar dreams also call for special attention; biblical examples include Joseph's parallel dreams suggesting that his brothers were going to worship him (the sun, the moon and 11 stars bowed down to him and his brother's sheaves of grain bowed down to his sheaves; Gen 37:6–10) and Pharaoh's two similar dreams of the coming famine (seven fat cows and seven lean cows, and seven fat ears of corn and seven lean ears of corn; Gen 41:1–7).

external verification (because they are dependent on the grace of the Sovereign Lord), but these examples raise the possibility of *asking* God for some external confirmation of a visionary message, particularly since this practice also has biblical precedents. Most notably, when Gideon was commissioned in a visitation to deliver Israel from the hand of Median, he asked the angel to "show me a sign that it is you who speak with me" (Judg 6:17) and the angel obliged and with his staff burned up the food he was offered (v. 21). Later, Gideon asked the Lord for a further sign:

> In order to see whether you will deliver Israel by my hand, as you have said, I am going to lay a fleece of wool on the threshing floor; if there is dew on the fleece alone, and it is dry on all the ground, then I shall know that you will deliver Israel by my hand, as you have said.
>
> (vv. 36–37)

And even after God had done what Gideon asked for, Gideon still felt the need to double-check:

> Do not let your anger burn against me, let me speak one more time; let me, please, make trial with the fleece just once more; let it be dry only on the fleece, and on all the ground let there be dew.
>
> (v. 39)

Again, God granted this verification request, as he also did in another high-profile biblical example, King Hezekiah's request for a sign to prove the truth of the message he had received through the Prophet Isaiah (reported in the Bible as many as three times: Isa 38: 7–8, 22; 2 Kgs 20:8–11; 2 Chr 32:24):

> Hezekiah said to Isaiah, "What shall be the sign that the Lord will heal me, and that I shall go up to the house of the Lord on the third day?" Isaiah said, "This is the sign to you from the Lord, that the Lord will do the thing that he has promised: the shadow has now advanced ten intervals; shall it retreat ten intervals?" Hezekiah answered, "It is normal for the shadow to lengthen ten intervals; rather let the shadow retreat ten intervals." The prophet Isaiah cried to the Lord; and he brought the shadow back the ten intervals, by which the sun had declined on the dial of Ahaz.
>
> (2 Kgs 20:8–11)

We also find further references to the external validation of vision in the Scriptures. In his epistles, Paul mentions the need to test prophecy twice: "Do not despise the words of prophets, but test everything" (1 Thess 5:20–21), and "Let two or three prophets speak, and let the others weigh what is said" (1 Cor 14:29). Although these verses do not offer any specific detail of how the external testing should proceed and who should be involved in performing it,[56] because the context of the second passage concerns the whole congregation, the required weighing process appears to be the collective responsibility of the whole church.[57] One consideration that can be raised to qualify this assumption is a point made by Leon Morris amongst others, namely that elsewhere Paul speaks about a particular spiritual gift specifically aimed at distinguishing between spirits (1 Cor 12:10), which would make it logical for certain people to specialise in exercising discernment.[58] However, even if this was a common practice in the early church, Paul did not emphasise it but left it to the whole congregation of believers to regulate the testing process.

An external verification method for visions that follows the same principles as the congregational sifting of prophecy is for the visionary to have a spiritual advisor, guide or director, who "is to be a co-discerner, to help us to interpret what God is saying to us."[59] This is, for example, a key element in Ignatian spirituality (see next chapter), where guides are seen as indispensable aids for identifying any deception or movement (i.e. fruit) within the retreatant's spiritual journey.[60] In his book-length discussion of private revelations, Groeschel specifically underlines this requirement:

> I have deliberately put beyond the scope of this book any real advice or counsel for those who think they have received a private revelation. Because of the danger of self-delusion, people in this situation need a director and not a book. The following few suggestions are given not to substitute for direction and wise counsel but to serve more as a caution.[61]

Arguably, the most elaborate method for the external evaluation of vision involves *institutional testing protocols* (ecclesiastical approbations) by established church communities. A series of controversies over the prophecies of mystics in the 14th century led the church to lay down formalised guidelines for distinguishing between true and false visions, adopting a rather sceptical attitude,[62] and, as Newman explains, in the 18th century the would-be Pope Benedict XIV published an influential treatise in which he submitted that even those private revelations that have been approved by the church

---

56 Fee, *God's Empowering Presence*, 171.
57 See e.g. Blomberg, *1 Corinthians*, 278–279; Fee, *God's Empowering Presence*, 252–253; Grudem, *Gift of Prophecy*, 57; Soards, *1 Corinthians*, 298.
58 Morris, *1 Corinthians*, 191. Thiselton (*1 Corinthians*, 1141) cites some scholarly opinions equating the "others" primarily with elders and church leaders.
59 Green, *Opening to God*, 56.
60 See e.g. English, *Spiritual Freedom*, 183.
61 Groeschel, *Reported Revelations*, 121.
62 Fraeters, "Vision/Vision," 188.

should be seen merely as a matter for individual judgment.[63] Currently, the most detailed protocol in existence is the Catholic church's 1987 *Norms regarding the manner of proceeding in the discernment of presumed apparitions or revelations*,[64] which contains guidelines for bishops for discerning private revelation (including vision) and which is centred around the three main aspects discussed earlier, the recipients, the content and the fruits of the vision. It is noteworthy, however, that according to Rahner, even such an ecclesiastical approbation is not infallible but pronounces only that the revelation "*can* show good grounds for human credibility and does not contradict the deposit of faith"[65] (emphasis added).

Illustration: was Eliphaz's dream in the Book of Job an authentic vision?

The Book of Job contains an extended vision report placed in a key position – at the beginning of the dispute between Job and his friends – which has a considerable impact on the whole of the subsequent discussion. The recipient of the vision, Eliphaz, accepts it as divine communication and shares it with Job as an important element of his overall argument. Despite the fact that his argument was ultimately rejected by God himself at the end of the book and that several concerns have been raised both about the form and the content of this vision over the centuries, the majority view in theology has been that Eliphaz's night-time vision describes an angelic visitation that conveys a divine message. This vision report thus lends itself to scrutiny through applying the verification principles discussed earlier. On the basis of this analysis, it will be proposed that the traditional mainstream interpretation has been misconstrued and that the spirit appearing to Eliphaz represents an agenda contrary to God's purposes. This alternative reading also provides a possible explanation of the age-old dilemma of why the seemingly righteous and Scripture-based arguments of Job's friends were rejected by God.[66] (For a more detailed analysis, see Chapter 5 of my book on *Progressive Creation and the Struggles of Humanity in the Bible.*[67])

Setting the scene

The story of the Book of Job is well known: the prologue starts with a conflict between God and his adversary, described there as the *śāṭān* ("accuser,"

---

63 Newman, "Medieval Visionary Culture," 42.
64 Sacred Congregation for the Doctrine of the Fait, *Norms Regarding Discernment.*
65 Rahner, *Visions and Prophecies*, 83.
66 There is general agreement that on the surface Eliphaz and his companions seem to be saying all the right things, sometimes even quoting well-known wisdom statements; for example, Andersen (*Job*, 98) states that "It is hard to find any proposition in the book which is not to some extent correct, taken in isolation," and Barth (*Church Dogmatics*, 453) contends that the friends "unquestionably speak good, earnest, and religious words."
67 Dörnyei, *Progressive Creation*, 140–151; 164–169.

equated in the Christian tradition with Satan[68]), when the latter questions the integrity of humankind, even that of Job, the most righteous man on earth. By doing so, the *śāṭān* expresses doubts about God's own testimony about Job and, more generally, about the soundness of God's created order. He then orchestrates a series of trials to test Job's integrity: first, Job's material possessions are destroyed, his children are killed and a horrible disease is inflicted on him; second, his wife makes an appeal to him to curse God and die; and third, three good friends arrive to comfort him and as part of their discussion they attempt to convince him that he is in the wrong and that his "theology" is flawed. This last trial constitutes by far the longest section of the book and it is also marked by a change from prose to poetry. Finally, in the epilogue, we learn that God sides with Job and restores his fortunes.

The current focus is on the very beginning of the poetic dispute between Job and his friends (Chapter 3), when the most senior of Job's visitors, Eliphaz, begins his response to Job's plea. First he strikes a conciliatory tone by emphasising that Job has played an exemplary role in the past by supporting people and building up the weak, and urging him not to be impatient. His initial advice seems fittingly righteous: fear God and trust him that "the integrity of your ways" (4:6) will bring you redemption. In v. 12, however, Eliphaz abruptly changes tack and presents a message he has received in a nocturnal vision, implying that this has provided his spiritual foundation:

> Now a word came stealing to me,
>   my ear received the whisper of it.
> Amid thoughts from visions of the night,
>   when deep sleep falls on mortals,
> dread came upon me, and trembling,
>   which made all my bones shake.
> A spirit glided past my face;
>   the hair of my flesh bristled.
> It stood still,
>   but I could not discern its appearance.
> A form was before my eyes;
>   there was silence, then I heard a voice:
> "Can mortals be righteous before God?
>   Can human beings be pure before their Maker?
> Even in his servants he puts no trust,
>   and his angels he charges with error;
> how much more those who live in houses of clay,
>   whose foundation is in the dust,
>   who are crushed like a moth.

68 However, the word *śāṭān* always appears in Job with the definite article in the Hebrew text, which likely indicates that it was not used as a proper name but rather in reference to someone having a descriptive title.

> Between morning and evening they are destroyed;
>   they perish forever without any regarding it.
> Their tent-cord is plucked up within them,
>   and they die devoid of wisdom."
>
> (Job 4:12–21)

The inconsistency between the reasonable start and the message of the subsequent vision has not escaped commentators, and several attempts have
been made to "correct" or explain away the visionary passage, for example
by detecting powerful irony in it,[69] by arguing that the text is written in such
ambiguous Hebrew that it is impossible to deduce a single meaning,[70] by
claiming that not all of the cited text is from God,[71] or – to take the most
radical but widely accepted solution (usually referred to as the "Tur-Sinai
and Ginsberg hypothesis") – by suggesting that the vision was actually given
to Job rather than to Eliphaz, and it was due to a redactional or copying
error that it is now mistakenly attributed to Eliphaz.[72]

The recipient of the vision

Eliphaz meets the requirements of a reliable source: he is presented as a person of high standing who genuinely worships God, and who, as a member
of the Wise, speaks from within the mainstream wisdom tradition.[73] This
lends credibility to his account, as does the frank reporting of the ambiguous
details of the apparition and of his own psychological reaction. As a result,
neither Job nor the other two friends question the source of the message,
and as mentioned earlier, most commentators in the past have accepted what
Eliphaz implies (although never explicitly states), namely that the spirit he
encountered was God's messenger.[74]

The content of the vision

Eliphaz admits about the spirit messenger that he "could not discern its
appearance" (4:16), indicating that he was aware of a degree of ambiguity

---

69 E.g. Clines, *Job 1–20*, 133; Habel, *Job*, 121–122; Janzen, *Job*, 73; Whybray, *Job*, 42.
70 Harding, "Spirit of Deception," 166.
71 E.g. Clines (*Job 1–20*, 133–134) regards v. 17 alone as the divine word of revelation in Elip-
    haz' s vision.
72 For a description of this view, see Ginsberg et al., "Job," 352; Greenstein, " 'On My Skin
    and in My Flesh,' " 66.
73 E.g. Ellison *Job*, 590.
74 In the most detailed analysis of Eliphaz's vision to date, Ken Brown (*Vision in Job 4*, 12)
    summarises that treating the vision as unproblematic has been "by far the most common
    approach in early modern commentaries, still regularly affirmed up to the present."

inherent to the situation.[75] Yet, it appears that the powerful signs accompanying the visitation were sufficient to convince him to attribute the message to God, which is consistent with the point made earlier regarding the convincing (and potentially deceiving) power of the symptoms of a religious experience. However, how can we explain the fact that readers of this report over the centuries, who have *not* been exposed to the full sensual experience of the apparition, did not become more suspicious? One reason, undoubtedly, has been the respectable context in which the report appears, a sacred book of the Bible. Furthermore, a review of the literature does show that many commentators have found certain details of the scene sinister, unusual and even weird:

- It is unlike other prophetic accounts of visions described in the Bible that there is no clear identification of the source of a divine message.[76] Therefore, Ash is right to conclude that "Eliphaz may imply that this is supernatural and therefore authoritative, but the author of the book subverts that claim and makes us suspect that something less positive is going on here."[77]
- Several commentators have noticed the eclectic nature of the components of the scene; Whybray, for example, finds that the details "seem to have been collected from a variety of sources,"[78] and according to Habel, the "bizarre collage of disparate allusions borders on a parody of traditional modes of revelation. Probable allusions to various revelatory traditions are deliberately brought into a clever juxtaposition of unlikely associations."[79] Thus, the vision report is rather *manufactured* in nature, almost as if it had been assembled to produce maximum impact on the receiver.[80]

---

75 The ambiguity of the source is also reflected by the discourse itself, because the text deliberately leaves some uncertainty in this respect by not specifying a definite subject in v. 16. Habel (*Job*, 128) sums up the scholarly consensus as follows: "The identity of the apparition is never revealed; the message alone is recorded. . . . The poet leaves Eliphaz – and us – floundering in wonder as to the source of the voice he hears." Newsom ("Job: Introduction," 378) agrees: "Eliphaz's choice of terms in the last part of the verse thus intimates but never explicitly claims that the apparition is a manifestation of God."
76 See e.g. Ash, *Job*, 106; Hartley, *Job*, 111.
77 Ash, *Job*, 106.
78 Whybray, *Job*, 43.
79 Habel, *Job*, 121. As he continues, "An anonymous word steals in, a vague sound is snatched, a nightmare intrudes on a deep sleep, a terror confronts the sleeper, a whirlwind makes him shiver, a veiled apparition is seen, something unknown stands before him, and finally a voice is heard after an ominous hush. The oracle received has no identified origin and is delivered by no known messenger. Eliphaz's message is a faint sound uttered by a fleeting spectre" (pp. 121–122).
80 As Brown (*Vision in Job 4*, 98) summarises, "Blending language and imagery from a vast array of distinct and often conflicting traditions, its every verse takes language that elsewhere reflects genuine revelatory activity, and twists it into something novel and unsettling."

- There is a degree of eeriness in the way Eliphaz refers to the amorphous presence that visits him, describing its coming with the word "stealing" and not hiding the dread it evoked in him, causing him to tremble and his body hair to bristle.[81] While such paralysing fear may not be indicative of anything unorthodox about the spirit – since the Bible records several occasions when humans feel terror in the presence of the numinous (e.g. Gen 15:12) – what is conspicuous here by its absence is some form of reassurance or encouragement along the customary "Fear not!" pattern (e.g. Gen 15:1; Judg 6:23; Dan 10:12) or at least a reassuring self-identification of the messenger.[82]

Given the above peculiarities, why did commentators still opt for accepting the scene as a divine visitation? Arguably, they came to this conclusion with hindsight, after the content of the message of the vision was seen to be delivering *bona fide* wisdom teaching.[83] However, a closer reading of the passage raises doubts about the orthodoxy of the content of what is actually communicated. To start with, most commentators remark on the *banality* of the spirit's first utterance: "Can mortals be righteous before God?" (4:17). Andersen sums up the general mood when he states, "After such a build-up, we expect to hear a revelation, not a truism. . . . The thing is so obviously impossible, that the banality makes Eliphaz sound pretentious."[84] There is clearly something amiss, and indeed, if we consider closely what the spirit actually says, we find that two aspects of the message are rather incompatible with established wisdom principles:

- While the primary focus of traditional wisdom teaching is on the nature of proper moral and religious conduct, this is not the tenor of the spirit's message in 4:17–21. Here he condemns the human race *en bloc*, without separating the righteous/wise from the wicked/foolish and without offering any links between good conduct and well-being in an attempt to show ways to remedy human sinfulness. That is, while biblical wisdom teaching does indeed condemn human sinfulness, Fyall correctly points out that it also "calls attention to the remedy and provides the strength to carry it out."[85] The spirit's message, in

---

81 According to Pope (*Job*, 36), "This passage is one of the most uncanny in the OT. The poet toys in poetic fancy with the dread effect of contact with the divine." Ash (*Job*, 106) compares the scene to a "horror movie."

82 See Fyall, *Job*, 147; Paul, "Experience of Eliphaz," 115.

83 Gordis's (*Job*, 41) summary represents well this interpretation: "Eliphaz then describes a revelation from on high that has brought him new insight: all men are imperfect in the eyes of God; therefore, even the suffering of the righteous has its justification. In view of these two great truths it is foolish for Job to lose patience and surrender his faith in the divine government of the world."

84 Andersen, *Job*, 114; see also Whybray, *Job*, 42; Ash, *Job*, 106.

85 Fyall, *Job*, 147.

contrast, emphasises only the absolute worthlessness and insignificance of humans.

- The spirit provides a curious justification for human worthlessness. Rather than focusing on the sinfulness of human nature, the main reason being offered is an *a fortiori* argument in the rhetorical sense: by contrasting immortal heavenly beings and inferior humans "whose foundation is in the dust" (4:19), the spirit argues that when even angels fall short of the mark in God's eyes, how much more so must this be true of human mortals.[86] Given that this message actually comes from a spiritual being, that is, a member of the group reported to be wanting in God's eyes, it is possible to identify a sense of bitterness behind the spirit's words along the lines of "If even the likes of myself are not good enough for God, how dare you think that you, a mere mortal, stand a chance?"

In sum, the spirit-carrier of the message is unlike God's angels in the Bible who visited humans on divine missions, and not only does the content of the message not convey traditional wisdom teaching but it also appears to represent the same agenda as the *śāṭān* did in the prologue of the book, a total lack of trust in the integrity of humanity.

The consequences of the vision

What was the fruit of the vision? Did it build up and encourage Eliphaz, and did the sharing of the vision report with Job make the latter feel consoled and closer to God? Exactly the opposite happened. The persuasive content of the spirit's words, accompanied by the sinister manner of their delivery, achieved its intended purpose of distorting Eliphaz's initially righteous stance. This is confirmed by the fact that a few verses later we read a reiteration of the *śāṭān*'s fundamental belief in human worthlessness, this time already paraphrased in Eliphaz's own words (5:6–7), and then, as a reflection of the extent to which Eliphaz adopted the stance of the nocturnal vision, in his second speech he delivers the same message again only in an even harsher manner, also reiterating the *a fortiori* argument (15:14–16).[87]

Finally, given this by now fully internalised belief in human worthlessness, it comes as no surprise that in his third and final speech Eliphaz reiterates this position one more time (22:2–5). We should note at this point that Eliphaz is presented by the text as the highest status person among Job's friends: he speaks first to Job and later God addresses him on behalf of his

---

86 See Whybray, *Job*, 43.
87 The language Eliphaz uses to dismiss humans, with words such as "abominable" and "corrupt," is unusually strong and emotive, suggesting to Newsom ("Job: Introduction," 450) an "almost visceral revulsion."

two companions. Therefore, the tenor of this speech sets the overall tone of how the friends' discussion with Job progresses; this is evidenced by the fact that in the last recorded statement by any of Job's friends, Bildad repeats Eliphaz's central doctrine of human worthlessness (25:4–6).[88]

In sum, the spirit's message of human worthlessness is reiterated by Job's friends as many as four times, including in the last recorded statement by any of the friends, demonstrating the extent to which the message, instilled in their thinking through a nocturnal vision, has infiltrated their whole mindset. As a result, they ended up, in effect, in the same camp as the *śāṭān*, and indeed, the way Job perceived their approach was not unlike the *śāṭān*'s disposition towards Job and humankind in general:

> How long will you torment me,
>   and break me in pieces with words?
> These ten times you have cast reproach upon me;
>   are you not ashamed to wrong me?
> . . . you magnify yourselves against me,
>   and make my humiliation an argument against me.
>   (19:2–3, 5)

External verification

We have seen that despite the eerie, fabricated nature of the visitation scene and the absence of any identified source or known messenger, Eliphaz accepted the vision as divine in origin. This instilled in him a doctrine of human worthlessness, which profoundly shaped both the tenor and the direction of his and his friends' arguments, thereby adding to Job's torments and temptation to turn against God. As a highly unique feature in the Bible, at the end of the book God responds to Job's plea in two long speeches, following which he explicitly sides with Job in his dispute with his friends, and tells Eliphaz: "My wrath is kindled against you and against your two friends; for you have not spoken of me what is right, as my servant Job has" (Job 42:7). This comes very close to an external verification, provided by God, the ultimate source of any divine vision.

Concluding remarks

Having submitted Eliphaz's vision report to an authentication exercise, it appears that the apparition did not originate from God but was part of a deception planted by God's spiritual opposition, most likely by the *śāṭān*

---

88 Besides its unequivocal blanket condemnation of humanity, the striking feature of this passage – similar to Eliphaz's second speech – is the strongly reviling figures of speech Bildad uses to characterize mankind: "maggots" and "worms." Clines (*Job 21–37*, 633) concludes that in comparing humans to unclean animals that are associated with decay and death, "Bildad is nothing if not brutal."

himself. This is admittedly a minority view,[89] but some scholars have pursued a similar train of argument,[90] and in a recent paper for example, Mart-Jan Paul has also proposed that "it seems likely that a negative or demonic spirit (related to Satan) tried to follow up the negative works of the first chapter."[91] The analysis was presented in detail to illustrate the complexity of trying to come to a clear-cut decision about the authenticity of a private visionary experience, particularly when deliberate deception might also be involved. The lasting ambiguity about Eliphaz's nocturnal vision illustrates well why vision interpretations can never offer cast-iron truths, and explains, for example, why even a detailed church protocol for discernment – the Catholic church's guidelines discussed earlier – will only talk about probabilities rather than certainties.

Summary

The reason why the authentication of vision is a serious matter is that vision itself is a serious matter, which can have an enormous impact on the life of both individuals and whole church communities. It was shown in this chapter that not only is vision vulnerable to unintended distortion and conscious abuse, but that its inherent vulnerability can also be capitalised on by spiritual forces which are not acting under God's authority. Accordingly, we have seen that even venerated Christian visionaries have been found to introduce erroneous elements into their vision reports over the past two millennia, and some of them actually lived in dread of delusion. The second half of the chapter presented several possible criteria and procedures that can be utilised to good effect to discern errors and deception in a vision, without denying the fact that these will always leave some room for doubt. An illustration of this latter point was offered in the form of a detailed analysis of one rather ambiguous biblical vision report, Eliphaz's dream in the Book of Job. It was argued that this contains a "false visitation" despite the fact that both the biblical recipient of the vision, Eliphaz, and the majority of the commentators of the text throughout the centuries have accepted it as coming from God.

Notwithstanding the fact that visionary experiences may never be completely safe against abuse, the Bible consistently portrays prophetic vision as one of the most valuable spiritual activities; and indeed, although the biblical authors repeatedly speak about the dangers of false prophecy, there is no recommendation in the Scriptures that we should ban or avoid prophecy to avert this danger. Accordingly, several theologians have insisted that vision must not be sidelined, because it forms an integral part of the Christian faith. Thus, given that humans are hard-wired to experience mental

89 E.g. Brown (*Vision in Job 4*, 12) insists that "the claim that the friends are portrayed as mouthpieces for Satan is not plausible."
90 E.g. Fyall, *Job*, 37; Janzen, *Job*, 73.
91 Paul, "Experience of Eliphaz," 120.

imagery, it has been argued in this chapter that the real issue is not so much *whether* we should engage with vision as *how* we can ensure that the human faculty of vision is used to good effect. Jesus instructed his disciples that they should "be wise as serpents and innocent as doves" (Matt 10:16), and the conclusion of the discussion in this chapter has been that exercising wisdom concerning vision through carefully examining the recipient, the content and the fruit of a visionary message, combined with some form of external verification, *can* ensure that visionary practices are as secure and reliable as most other Christian activities.

References

Andersen, Francis I. 1976. *Job: An Introduction and Commentary*. Leicester: Inter-Varsity Press.

Arnold, William T. 1996. "Visions." In *Evangelical Dictionary of Biblical Theology*, edited by Walter A. Elwell, 802–03. Grand Rapids, MI: Baker Books.

Ash, Christopher. 2014. *Job: The Wisdom of the Cross*. Wheaton, IL: Crossway.

Ashley, Timothy R. 1993. *The Book of Numbers*. New International Commentary on the Old Testament. Grand Rapids, MI: Eerdmans.

Augustine of Hippo. *On the Literal Meaning of Genesis* (in: *On Genesis*). Translated by Edmund Hill. New York: New City Press, 415/2002.

Aune, David E. 1988. "Ecstasy." In *The International Standard Bible Encyclopedia, Revised*, edited by Geoffrey W. Bromiley, 14–16. Grand Rapids, MI: Eerdmans.

Barth, Karl. 1961. *Church Dogmatics IV/3.1: Jesus Christ, the True Witness*. Edinburgh: T & T Clark.

Blomberg, Craig L. 1994. *1 Corinthians*. Grand Rapids, MI: Zondervan.

Boyd, Gregory A. 2004. *Seeing Is Believing: Experience Jesus through Imaginative Prayer*. Grand Rapids, MI: Baker Books.

Brown, Ken. 2015. *The Vision in Job 4 and Its Role in the Book: Reframing the Development of the Joban Dialogues*. Tübingen: Mohr Siebeck.

Buber, Martin. 1949/1985. *The Prophetic Faith*. New York: Collier.

Carson, D. A. 2010. "Matthew." In *The Expositor's Bible Commentary: Matthew – Mark (Revised Edition)*, edited by Tremper III Longman and David E. Garland, 23–671. Grand Rapids, MI: Zondervan.

Clines, David J. 1989. A. *Job 1–20*. Dallas, Tex.: Word Books.

Clines, David J. 2006. A. *Job 21–37*. Dallas, Tex.: Word Books.

Dörnyei, Zoltán. 2018. *Progressive Creation and Humanity's Struggles in the Bible: A Canonical Narrative Interpretation*. Eugene, OR: Pickwick.

Dunn, James D. G. 1997. "Biblical Concepts of Revelation." In *Divine Revelation*, edited by Paul Avis, 1–22. Eugene, OR: Wipf and Stock.

Elliott, Dyan. 2012. "Raptus/Rapture." In *The Cambridge Companion to Christian Mysticism*, edited by Amy Hollywood and Patricia Zoltán Beckman, 189–99. Cambridge: Cambridge University Press.

Ellison, H. L. 1996. "Book of Job." In *New Bible Dictionary*, edited by I. Howard Marshall, A. R. Millard, J. I. Packer and D. J. Wiseman, 589–90. Downers Grove, IL: InterVarsity Press.

English, John J. 1995. *Spiritual Freedom: From an Experience of the Ignatian Exercises to the Art of Spiritual Guidance*. 2nd ed. Chicago: Loyola University Press.

Fee, Gordon D. 1994. *God's Empowering Presence: The Holy Spirit in the Letters of Paul*. Peabody, MA: Hendrickson.

Fraeters, Veerle. 2012. "Visio/Vision." In *The Cambridge Companion to Christian Mysticism*, edited by Amy Hollywood and Patricia Zoltán Beckman, 178–88. Cambridge: Cambridge University Press.

Futrell, John Carroll. 1970. "Ignatian Discernment." *Studies in the Spirituality of Jesuits* 2, no. 2: 47–88.

Fyall, Robert S. 2002. *Now My Eyes Have Seen You: Images of Creation and Evil in the Book of Job*. Leicester: Apollos.

Gallagher, Timothy M. 2008. *Meditation and Contemplation: An Ignatian Guide to Praying with Scripture*. New York: Crossroad.

Ginsberg, Harold Louis, Mayer I. Gruber, Theodore Friedman, Judith R. Baskin, Haïm Z'ew Hirschberg, and Bathja Bayer. 2007. "Book of Job." In *Encyclopaedia Judaica*, edited by Michael Berenbaum and Fred Skolnik, 341–59. Detroit, MI: Macmillan Reference.

Gordis, Robert. 1978. *The Book of Job: Commentary, New Translation and Special Studies*. New York: The Jewish Theological Seminary of America.

Green, Thomas H. 2006. *Opening to God: A Guide to Prayer*. Rev. ed. Notre Dame, IN: Ave Maria Press.

Green, Thomas H. 2009. *When the Well Runs Dry: Prayer Beyond the Beginnings*. Rev. ed. Notre Dame, IN: Ave Maria Press.

Greenstein, Edward L. 2007. "'On My Skin and in My Flesh': Personal Experience as a Source of Knowledge in the Book of Job." In *Bringing the Hidden to Light: The Process of Interpretation: Studies in Honor of Stephen A. Geller*, edited by Kathryn F. Kravitz and Diane M. Sharon, 63–77. Winona Lake, IN: Eisenbrauns.

Groeschel, Benedict J. 1993. *A Still, Small Voice: A Practical Guide on Reported Revelations*. San Francisco: Ignatius.

Grudem, Wayne. 2000. *The Gift of Prophecy in the New Testament and Today*. Rev. ed. Wheaton, IL: Crossway.

Habel, Norman C. 1985. *The Book of Job: A Commentary*. London: SCM.

Hamon, Jane. 2016. *Dreams and Visions: Understanding and Interpreting God's Messages to You*. Rev. ed. Minneapolis, MN: Chosen Books.

Harding, James E. 2005. "A Spirit of Deception in Job 4:15? Interpretive Indeterminacy and Eliphaz's Vision." *Biblical Interpretation* 13, no. 2: 137–66.

Hart, David Bentley. 2017. *The New Testament: A Translation*. New Haven, CT: Yale University Press.

Hartley, John E. 1988. *The Book of Job*. Grand Rapids, MI: Eerdmans.

Hultgård, Anders. 1982. "Ecstasy and Vision." *Scripta Instituti Donneriani Aboensis* 11: 187–200.

Janzen, J. Gerald. 1985. *Job: A Bible Commentary for Teaching and Preaching*. Atlanta, GA: John Knox.

Johnson, Luke Timothy. 1998. *Religious Experience in Earliest Christianity: A Missing Dimension in New Testament Studies*. Minneapolis, MN: Fortress.

Kaiser, Walter C. 1996. "False Prophets." In *Evangelical Dictionary of Biblical Theology*, edited by Walter A. Elwell, 242–43. Grand Rapids, MI: Baker.

Lonsdale, David. 2000. *Eyes to See, Ears to Hear: An Introduction to Ignatian Spirituality*. London: Darton, Longman and Todd.

McGinn, Bernard. 2006. *The Essential Writings of Christian Mysticism*. New York: Modern Library.

McKane, William. 1986. *Jeremiah. Vol 1: Introduction and Commentary on Jeremiah I – Xxv*. Critical and Exegetical Commentary. Edinburgh: T & T Clark.

Morris, Leon. 1985. *1 Corinthians: An Introduction and Commentary*. Tyndale New Testament Commentaries 17. Downers Grove, IL: IVP Academic.

Newman, Barbara. 2005. "What Did It Mean to Say "I Saw"? The Clash between Theory and Practice in Medieval Visionary Culture." *Speculum* 80, no. 1: 1–43.

Newsom, Carol A. 1996. "The Book of Job: Introduction, Commentary, and Reflections." In *The New Interpreter's Bible*, edited by Leander E. Keck, 319–637. Nashville, TN: Abingdon.

Paul, Mart-Jan. 2016. "The Disturbing Experience of Eliphaz in Job 4: Divine or Demonic Manifestation?". In *Goochem in Mokum, Wisdom in Amsterdam: Papers on Biblical and Related Wisdom Read at the Fifteenth Joint Meeting of the Society for Old Testament Study and the Oudtestamentisch Werkgezelschap, Amsterdam July 2012*, edited by George J. Brooke and Pierre van Hecke, 108–20. Leiden: Brill.

Pope, Marvin H. 1965. *Job: Introduction, Translation, and Notes*. Garden City, NY: Doubleday.

Proudfoot, Wayne. 1985. *Religious Experience*. Berkeley, CA: University of California Press.

Rahner, Karl. 1963. *Visions and Prophecies*. Translated by Charles H. Henkey and Richard Strachan. Freiburg: Herder.

Sacred Congregation for the Doctrine of the Faith. 1978. *Norms Regarding the Manner of Proceeding in the Discernment of Presumed Apparitions or Revelations*. Vatican. www.vatican.va/roman_curia/congregations/cfaith/documents/rc_con_cfaith_doc_19780225_norme-apparizioni_en.html.

Seal, David. 2016. "Prophetic Ecstasy in the Ancient Near East." In *The Lexham Bible Dictionary*, edited by John D. Barry, David Bomar, Derek R. Brown, Rachel Klippenstein, Douglas Mangum, Carrie Sinclair Wolcott, Lazarus Wentz, Elliot Ritzema and Wendy Widder. Bellingham, WA: Lexham Press.

Shantz, Colleen. 2009. *Paul in Ecstasy: The Neurobiology of the Apostle's Life and Thought*. Cambridge: Cambridge University Press.

Soards, Marion L. 1999. *1 Corinthians*. Understanding the Bible. Grand Rapids, MI: Baker Books.

Sveshnikov, Sergei. 2009. *Imagine That: Mental Imagery in Roman Catholic and Eastern Orthodox Private Devotion*. North Charleston, SC: CreateSpace.

Swanson, James. 1997. *Dictionary of Biblical Languages with Semantic Domains: Hebrew (Old Testament)*. electronic ed. Oak Harbor, WA: Logos Research Systems.

Thiselton, Anthony C. 2000. *The First Epistle to the Corinthians: A Commentary on the Greek Text*. NIGTC. Grand Rapids, MI: Eerdmans.

Van Dam, Cornelis. 2012. "Divination, Magic." In *Dictionary of the Old Testament: Prophets*, edited by Mark J. Boda and Gordon J. McConville, 159–62. Downers Grove, IL: IVP Academic.

Whybray, R. Norman. 1998. *Job*. Sheffield: Sheffield Academic Press.

6   Cultivated vision, Ignatian spirituality and vision-led ministry

The previous chapter discussed how human strivings to generate vision may increase the chances of including subjective human elements in a divine message, thereby opening the vision up to potential error and even diabolical abuse. While these dangers are real and false prophets are described in the Bible to be able to cause serious damage, visionary practices have also been at the heart of pursuing a true relationship with God, and several respected theologians were cited earlier as urging the church not to "throw the baby out with the bathwater" by excluding divine vision from legitimate Christian life. In agreement with this inclusive stance, the current chapter presents two broad traditions that have utilised the notion of vision to good effect in enriching and energising Christian conduct and ministry, following two different approaches. The first concerns the pursuit of *cultivated vision*, that is, consciously adding mental imagery to prayer or the reading of Scripture; various forms of this approach have been applied in established Christian practices over the centuries, from gospel meditation and Ignatian spirituality to imaginative prayer. The second approach concerns the harnessing of the motivational power of an envisaged ideal future state, not unlike the use of vision in the business world (discussed in Chapter 2). This practice has become a central element within the discussions of contemporary Christian leadership and church growth, and in fact, the vast majority of the contemporary Christian literature on vision focuses on this theme.

Cultivated vision and Ignatian spirituality

It was mentioned in Chapter 5 that starting in the Middle Ages there was a growing tendency to facilitate visionary experiences by means of various intensive meditative techniques. As a result, according to Newman, *cultivated visions* became more common than spontaneous ones.[1] The main form of this practice was *gospel meditation*[2] (also called "scripted

---

1 Newman, "Medieval Visionary Culture," 3.
2 See Karnes, *Imagination*, 8.

vision"[3]), which involved the conscious visualisation of what was read (or recalled) in the Scriptures. We shall begin our exploration of cultivated vision with examining the main characteristics of this practice and then describe a highly influential spiritual approach that was introduced by St. Ignatius of Loyola in the middle of the 16th century – usually referred to as *Ignatian spirituality* – which elevated gospel meditation to a new level of sophistication by embedding it into a coherent programme of spiritual growth. This approach is still widely practised in the Jesuit order, and it has also had a broader influence that reached beyond the Roman Catholic church through the promotion of *imaginative prayer*, which will be the final theme addressed within the subject of cultivated vision.

Gospel meditation

Rowland explains that in gospel meditation "the words become the catalyst for the exercise of imagination as text is taken up and infuses the imagination."[4] Because of the growing interest in this practice, the late Middle Ages (14th-15th centuries) saw the publication and proliferation of visionary scripts aimed at helping a wider audience – even uneducated laypeople – to gain access to visionary experience.[5] The most famous of these works, *Meditations on the Life of Christ*[6] (hence, *Meditations*), was written in the 14th century by a Franciscan friar in Italy,[7] and was rendered into many vernacular translations in Europe, such as Nicholas Love's *Mirror of the Blessed Life of Jesus Christ* in Middle English.[8] The *Meditations* was addressed to a Poor Clare nun, and it included explicit instructions on how to use the script;[9] according to the Prologue, "if you wish to profit you must be present at the same things that it is related that Christ did and said, joyfully and rightly, leaving behind all other cares and anxieties."[10] Thus, paraphrased in contemporary language, the author's advice is to "relax and imagine that you are an eyewitness," which makes the text, in effect, extensive Scripture-based guided imagery.[11]

---

3 See Newman, "Medieval Visionary Culture," 25.
4 Rowland, "Visionary Experience," 50.
5 Newman, "Medieval Visionary Culture," 6.
6 Ragusa and Green, *Meditation*.
7 Until the 19th century it was regarded as the work of the Franciscan theologian Bonaventure; for a recent detailed analysis of date and authorship, suggesting Jacobus de Sancto Geminianio as a possible author, see Tóth and Falvay, "New Light."
8 See Sargent, *Blessed Life of Jesus*.
9 Karnes (*Imagination*, 145) states that "Instructing its reader or hearer to meditate systematically on the events of Christ's life and often modelling meditations for her use, the text is the most self-conscious of medieval gospel meditations."
10 Ragusa and Green, *Meditation*, 5.
11 While such scripturally guided imageries became widely used in the Middle Ages, there are records of much earlier occurrences. For example, Ensley (*Visions*, 36) draws attention to a guided imagery presented by Cyril, Archbishop of Jerusalem, in the Prologue to his

Regarding its overall purpose, the *Meditations* describes itself as a "spiritual exercise,"[12] presenting the activity involved as "the most necessary and the most fruitful and the one that may lead to the highest level."[13] The author declares that "continuous contemplation of the life of Jesus Christ fortifies and steadies the intellect against trivial and transient things . . . against trials and adversity. . . [and against] enemies and vices."[14] Above all, through "continued meditation on His life the soul attains so much familiarity, confidence, and love that it will disdain and disregard other things and be exercised and trained as to what to do and what to avoid."[15] These extracts adequately summarise the stated value of imaginative meditation of the age.

Gospel meditation rested on a sound theological basis, since active remembrance of Jesus is a central biblical message. For example, during the Last Supper, Jesus specifically instructed his followers to remember his sacrificial death, which foregrounds and justifies any meditation on the Passion. We should note that the semantic domain of the Greek word for "remembrance" (*anamnesis*) used in the verses that describe the Eucharist (Luke 22:19 and 1 Corinthians 11:24) is broader than purely cognitive recollection, as it also includes a sense of the participatory act of "making the past present"[16] – indeed, the *TDNT* describes its meaning as the "reliving of vanished impressions by a definite act of will"[17] – which is in full harmony with the goals of gospel meditation.

We saw earlier when discussing transportation theory (in Chapter 2) that using scripted mental imagery may transport the reader into the alternative world of the text. It was consistent with this theory that medieval scholars – and most notably, the Franciscan theologian, Bonaventure (1221–1274) – proposed that by using the Scriptures as the basis of meditation, the meditant could embark on a meditative journey from Christ's humanity to his divinity – or as Karnes puts it, following a "trajectory from earth to

---

Catechetical Lectures (Par. 15) (www.ccel.org/ccel/schaff/npnf207.ii.iv.html): "Even now, I beseech you, lift up the eye of the mind: even now imagine the choirs of Angels, and God the Lord of all there sitting, and His Only-begotten Son sitting with Him on His right hand, and the Spirit present with them; and Thrones and Dominions doing service, and every man of you and every woman receiving salvation. Even now let your ears ring, as it were, with that glorious sound, when over your salvation the angels shall chant . . ."

12 Ragusa and Green, *Meditation*, 2.
13 Ibid.
14 Ibid., 2–3.
15 Ibid., 2.
16 E.g. Kelly, *Early Christian Doctrines*, 197; Spinks, *Eucharist*, 20; Thiselton, *Dictionary of Theology*, 551.
17 Behm, "Ἀνάμνησις," 348. O'Loughlin (*Eucharist*, 119) offers an expressive description of this sense of awareness: "By 'memory' we do not mean simply 'tales from long ago' or even 'our Story' but that profound awareness of reality which appreciates its origins and its ends. This awareness is the realization, in this moment as we eat, that we have an actual connection to a much larger reality."

heaven"[18] – thereby connecting with some aspects of transcendent reality.[19] After all, it is clearly stated in the Scriptures that Jesus is "the image of the invisible God" (Col 1:15) and "Whoever has seen me has seen the Father" (John 14:9; see also John 1:18). Imagining Jesus' earthly ministry simulates the experiences of those people who actually encountered Jesus in person in New Testament times, and as such, it can help one to perceive the divine revelation of God in the form of his Son.

In summary, according to Scripture, the Word became flesh (John 1:14), and therefore by meditating on the flesh – that is, on the life of Jesus – the meditant may in effect explore the divine Word. Bernard McGinn points out in this respect that several verses in John's Gospel (e.g. 1:18 and 14:8–9) insist that the only way by which one can "see" the divine Father is through his eternal Son,[20] and that it is this element which distinguishes Christian contemplation from other meditative approaches. This being the case, the practice of mentally visualising the incarnate Christ might allow a glimpse into heaven, which is why Karnes calls gospel meditation "an extension of Christ's gift of himself in the incarnation."[21] In fact, Karnes believes that Christ's life and passion were specifically intended for "mental commemoration,"[22] and the vivid experiences of various mystics documented over the centuries have evidenced that such mental commemoration can indeed lead to a sense of transcendent reality that can be as powerful as the reception of divine communication directly from heaven (which was the essence of biblical vision discussed in Chapter 4).

Centring the vision around Jesus' life and death within a scriptural framework goes a considerable way to safeguarding the content of the meditative practice.[23] Interestingly, we find explicit references to such safety concerns in a letter written by the renowned theologian and mystic, William of St. Thierry, as early as the middle of the 12th century:

> The best and safest reading matter and subject for meditation for the animal man, newly come to Christ, to train him in the interior life, is the outward actions of our Redeemer . . . so that the weak spirit which

18 Karnes, *Imagination*, 111.
19 As Karnes (*Imagination*, 112–113) later elaborates, "Bonaventure did not independently invent this conception of gospel meditations, but rather developed various comments made by his predecessors who had understood meditations, at least implicitly, as journeys to God. Making that journey explicit, he provided a concrete mechanism by which to accomplish it. That mechanism, in fact, is Bonaventure's defining innovation to the genre. In his hands, gospel meditation becomes a technical activity with an ambitious goal and a systematic method by which to reach it."
20 McGinn, *Christian Mysticism*, 311.
21 Karnes, *Imagination*, 144.
22 Ibid., 146.
23 Although the controversies in the Middle Ages indicated that even within a Scripture-based paradigm one can go to imaginative extremes that would be considered heretical.

is only able to think of material objects and properties may have something to which it can apply itself and cling with devout attention, as
befits its degree. Christ. . . . When the novice concentrates his powers
upon him, thinking of God in a human form, he does not wholly depart
from the truth. . . .[24]

Ignatian spirituality

St. Ignatius of Loyola, the founder of the Jesuit order, published a treatise in 1548 – entitled *Spiritual Exercises*[25] – that was intended to serve as
a manual for spiritual retreats. It offers structured guidelines for a Christian retreat divided into four weekly parts, focusing on various forms of
"examination of conscience, of meditation, of contemplation, of vocal and
mental prayer, and of other spiritual activities."[26] This work has exerted
enormous influence on believers over the past 500 years, reaching beyond
the Jesuit order and even the Catholic church, due to two crucial aspects of
the material:

- First, by drawing on the guided visual meditative techniques described
  in the previous section, it offers an intensive and personally engaging
  approach to strengthening one's relationship (or communion) with God
  within a framework that is theologically robust and which pays sufficient attention to avoiding the possibility of distortion discussed in
  Chapter 5.
- Second, it presents an explicit life-changing agenda by centring the
  material around the "Election," a term used by Ignatius to refer to a
  major choice or decision that the participants are encouraged to make
  during the course of the retreat.

We have seen earlier that the *Meditations on the Life of Christ* became
an international bestseller, and Ignatius's *Spiritual Exercises* takes the cultivated vision approach explored in that book to a new level of depth and
sophistication. Therefore, Boyd rightly characterises Ignatius as the person
"who most profoundly thought through the role of imagination in prayer
during the Middle Ages and Renaissance – and arguably in any other
period."[27] Let us examine more closely three aspects of Ignatian spirituality
that are particularly relevant to the treatment of vision in the current book:
the nature of its key component, "contemplation"; the discernment of spirits; and the motivational agenda of the "Election."

24 Cited in Sargent, "Introduction," xi.
25 Puhl, *The Spiritual Exercises of St Ignatius*; also available at http://spex.ignatianspiritual
   ity.com/SpiritualExercises/Puhl
26 *Spiritual Exercises*, Introductory Observations, 1.
27 Boyd, *Seeing Is Believing*, 92.

Ignatian contemplation

The term "contemplation," along with its counterpart, "meditation," has a specific meaning within the Ignatian paradigm: *contemplation* is the visionary element, referring to the use of the imagination in terms of mental imagery, and *meditation* complements contemplation by adding the cognitive aspect, that is, reasoned understanding. They represent the two foundational approaches to Ignatian prayer with Scripture, and they used to form the essence of medieval Scripture-oriented spirituality, with the Franciscan approach (discussed earlier regarding the *Meditations*) leaning towards the former and the Benedictine approach (particularly the "*Lectio Divina*") towards the latter.[28] The present focus will be on the process of contemplation, and we must note here Timothy Gallagher's caution that Ignatius used the term somewhat differently from the mystical connotation associated with his influential contemporary, John of the Cross: for John, contemplation signifies "infused, passive, mystical prayer," whereas for Ignatius, contemplation signifies "active imaginative participation in a Gospel event."[29]

One of the most effective recent ambassadors of Ignatian spirituality and contemplative prayer, Thomas Green, describes the essence of contemplation through using the scene of Jesus and the Samaritan woman at the well (John 4:1–42) as an illustration; because it would be difficult to offer a more expressive characterisation of the process, let us cite this explanation at some length:

> Contemplation involves imaginatively entering into the incident we are considering – being present at the event seeing it happen as if we were actually participants ourselves . . . and we seek to relive, not some movie, but the life of the Lord Jesus. In our example, we seek to be present at the well when Jesus meets the woman. Perhaps we are sitting beside him as she comes walking along the road. We notice his face (he is "weary"). We see what a woman looks like who has had five and a half husbands, and who is tired of having to come to the well day after day. We feel the heat of the noonday sun in this semitropical land. . . . And then Jesus speaks to this strange woman. We hear his words, note the tone of his voice, observe the surprised look on the face of the woman. We listen, and look, as their dialogue unfolds – and we imagine how we would have reacted had we been in the woman's place. Perhaps we share her puzzlement at Jesus' reference to living water. Perhaps, if we are lucky, we find ourselves involved in the conversation. . . . We may even, in our contemplation, find ourselves remaining at the well with Jesus, when the woman hurries off to town to tell the people – and

28 The Benedictine practice of "*Lectio Divina*" involves the meditative reading of the Bible and thereby engaging in a slow, thoughtful and reflective dwelling on Scripture.
29 Gallagher, *Meditation and Contemplation*, 11.

we may learn by experience what it means to have him tell us every-thing we have ever done.[30]

This example shows how the application of mental imagery in Ignatian imaginative contemplation tends to follow a three-step approach in relation to a gospel scene: "to see the persons," "to hear what they say" and "to observe what they do."[31] The exercise usually ends with directly engaging with Christ in some form, for example through a conversation. We shall return to contemplation when we discuss the notion of imaginative prayer in a separate section.

Discernment of the spirits

Ignatius was fully aware of the dangers of diabolical interference during contemplation, and discussed this matter in the *Spiritual Exercises* by con-trasting two spirits, the good spirit and the bad or evil spirit, with the former typically understood as the Holy Spirit, the latter as the devil. He character-ises the evil spirit as "proposing fallacious reasonings, subtleties, and con-tinual deceptions"[32] and even masquerading as the good spirit:

> It is a mark of the evil spirit to assume the appearance of an angel of light. He begins by suggesting thoughts that are suited to a devout soul, and ends by suggesting his own. For example, he will suggest holy and pious thoughts that are wholly in conformity with the sanctity of the soul. Afterwards, he will endeavour little by little to end by drawing the soul into his hidden snares and evil designs.[33]

As a response to these dangers, the *Spiritual Exercises* contains five com-ponents to safeguard the participants' spiritual experiences: (a) a recurring prayer structure; (b) a spiritual director/guide; (c) regular self-checks (called the "Examen"); (d) an elaborate system of describing two types of inner movements, "consolation" and "desolation," which act as spiritual ther-mometers; and (e) a foundation of humility and love. Let us examine these components more closely.

Recurring prayer. At the beginning of the *Exercises*, a preparatory prayer is prescribed: "In the preparatory prayer I will beg God our Lord for grace that all my intentions, actions, and operations may be directed purely to the praise and service of His Divine Majesty."[34] It is then specified in a special

---

30 Green, *Opening to God*, 103–104.
31 Gallagher, *Meditation and Contemplation*, 102; good examples of sets of these three steps are presented in *Spiritual Exercises* 106–109 and 114–116.
32 *Spiritual Exercises* 329.
33 Ibid., 332.
34 Ibid., 046.

note that this prayer "must always be made before *all* the contemplations and meditations"[35] (emphasis added). In this way, there is ongoing and comprehensive prayer coverage throughout the whole retreat.

Spiritual director/guide. The layer of protection provided by the prayer coverage is strengthened by the active presence of an experienced spiritual director/guide, who oversees every aspect of the retreat participants' spiritual development and who offers help to discern the spirits. For example, the seventh Introductory Observation states:

> If the director of the Exercises observes that the exercitant is in desolation and tempted, let him not deal severely and harshly with him, but gently and kindly. He should encourage and strengthen him for the future by exposing to him the wiles of the enemy of our human nature, and by getting him to prepare and dispose himself for the coming consolation.[36]

Examen. At the beginning of the first week of the retreat, the *Spiritual Exercises* prescribes two daily "Examinations of Conscience," usually referred to as "Examen," one around noon and the other at the end of the day.[37] These reviews involve a thorough self-examination of the retreatant's experiences and emotions since the last Examen, asking God to identify any mistakes or sinful behaviours, and then praying for forgiveness and healing. The following gives a flavour of the reflection process:

> When the enemy of our human nature has been detected and recognized by the trail of evil marking his course and by the wicked end to which he leads us, it will be profitable for one who has been tempted to review immediately the whole course of the temptation. . . . The purpose of this review is that once such an experience has been understood and carefully observed, we may guard ourselves for the future against the customary deceits of the enemy.[38]

The two key concepts within the Ignatian framework of the Examen are "consolation" and "desolation," and the special significance and implications of these concepts warrant a closer look at them. However, we should also note that although Ignatius provides specific guidelines for discernment in this respect, one may also have to "improvise and adjust because God works in each of us so uniquely."[39]

Consolation and desolation. The repeated self-reflection exercise of the Examen allows believers to become aware of what Ignatius calls the "motions of the soul," that is, inner movements of one's emotions; these in

---

35 Ibid., 049.
36 Ibid., 007.
37 Ibid., 024–026.
38 Ibid., 334.
39 O'Brien, *The Ignatian Adventure*, 115.

turn can be seen as indicators of whether one is on the right spiritual trajectory or not. This *phenomenological* approach to discernment thus assumes that our affective state reflects our spiritual health in a perceptible way, and the Ignatian system is unique in that it focuses on the *direction* of the emotional changes by specifying two trajectories, *consolation* and *desolation*. Ignatius describes consolation as follows:

> I call it consolation when an interior movement is aroused in the soul, by which it is inflamed with love of its Creator and Lord, and . . . when one sheds tears that move to the love of God, whether it be because of sorrow for sins, or because of the sufferings of Christ our Lord, or for any other reason that is immediately directed to the praise and service of God. Finally, I call consolation every increase of faith, hope, and love, and all interior joy that invites and attracts to what is heavenly and to the salvation of one's soul by filling it with peace and quiet in its Creator and Lord.[40]

Thus, consolation involves the perception of growth in any area related to the gifts and fruit of the Spirit (for more discussion of love, see the following component). As the quotation indicates, it is not equated exclusively with joy, because it can also occur amongst hardships and challenges if one feels that one's spirit is moving in the right direction. Desolation is the opposite of consolation as it involves moving away from God and is characterised by "darkness of soul, turmoil of spirit, inclination to what is low and earthly, restlessness rising from many disturbances and temptations which lead to want of faith, want of hope, want of love."[41] Accordingly, Ignatius concludes that in desolation the soul is "wholly slothful, tepid, sad, and separated, as it were, from its Creator and Lord."[42] People sometimes try to alleviate the discomfort of desolation through various "comfort" activities (e.g. eating, drinking) or pursuing distractions. It is important to note that, as George Aschenbrenner underlines, desolation is not usually "a loss of intellectual belief in God's providence; rather, as something much more subtle, the temptations tend toward a distrust of God that can take the heart out of hope and love."[43] The difference between consolation and desolation is illustrated by Ignatius with two contrasting images:

> In souls that are progressing to greater perfection, the action of the good angel is delicate, gentle, delightful. It may be compared to a drop of water penetrating a sponge. The action of the evil spirit upon such souls is violent, noisy, and disturbing. It may be compared to a drop of water falling upon a stone.[44]

---

40 *Spiritual Exercises*, 316.
41 Ibid.
42 Ibid.
43 Aschenbrenner, *Stretched for Greater Glory*, 172.
44 *Spiritual Exercises*, 335.

Foundation of humility and love. It was shown in Chapter 5 that while the Orthodox church tends to discourage the use of mental imagery in prayer, it accepts that divine vision may be authentic if it is steeped in repentance and humility (i.e. if it occurs within the context of the ongoing Jesus Prayer). Ignatius formulates a similar spiritual safeguard, the overall foundation of *humility* and *love,* and emphasises these elements recurrently in the *Spiritual Exercises.* Michael Ivens explains that the essence of Ignatius's notion of humility is "self-subjection," and continues, "Humility is in fact nothing other than the love of God, . . . a handing over oneself in trust, letting God be Lord of one's being."[45] He cites a retreatant who made the *Exercises* under Ignatius's guidance in 1538 and described the modes of humility as "kinds and degrees of the love of God, and of desiring to obey, imitate and serve his Divine Majesty."[46] The significance of love is then summarised by Ignatius as follows:

> The love that moves and causes one to choose must descend from above, that is, from the love of God, so that before one chooses he should perceive that the greater or less attachment for the object of his choice is solely because of His Creator and Lord.[47]

Pheme Perkins calls this principle the most important rule of spiritual discernment in Ignatius's work,[48] and we find in fact a whole exercise in the *Spiritual Exercises* focusing on "Contemplation to Attain the Love of God,"[49] which includes a prayer of total self-offering:

> Take, Lord, and receive all my liberty, my memory, my understanding, and my entire will, all that I have and possess. Thou hast given all to me. To Thee, O Lord, I return it. All is Thine, dispose of it wholly according to Thy will. Give me Thy love and Thy grace, for this is sufficient for me.[50]

Election

"Election" is a technical term within the English terminology of Ignatian spirituality, originating from the Spanish word *elección* used in the *Spiritual Exercises.* Although *elección* literally means "choice," Ignatius used it to refer to a fundamental, potentially life-changing decision that the retreat participants are encouraged to make about their future vocation, and the term "Election" is intended to reflect this special connotation. Some scholars

---

45 Ivens, *Understanding the Spiritual Exercises,* 123.
46 Ibid.
47 *Spiritual Exercises,* 184.
48 Perkins, *Ephesians,* 395.
49 *Spiritual Exercises,* 230–237.
50 Ibid., 234.

believe that the primary purpose of the *Spiritual Exercises* is centred around the Election,[51] while others consider the main objective to be the promotion of the retreatant's union with God through contemplation and meditation.[52] However, Election and communion with God need not to be placed in a contrasting position but can be understood to go hand in hand: Ignatius clearly states that "The love that moves and causes one to choose must descend from above, that is, from the love of God,"[53] and therefore the stronger the communion with God, the more accurate the discernment of God's intention for a person. As Rahner summarises, "The purpose of the meditations . . . is to discover the imperative in the life of Jesus that applies to me alone, and then to make the choice to carry it out in my life."[54]

Thus, Ignatius's *Spiritual Exercises* offers an integrated approach of promoting a cultivated vision of Jesus' life and motivating a transformation of the retreatant's life. The centrality of the latter is reflected by the fact that of all the Ignatian exercises, the Election is prepared with the greatest care,[55] with the *Exercises* offering a series of aids to facilitate the decision-making process. As Rahner concludes, "St. Ignatius wants the exercitant to stir up in himself the courage to make a binding choice that will truly affect his life, even if it is only in a very small matter."[56] What makes Ignatius's guidelines particularly relevant for the present discussion is that the prescribed principles and methods are not limited to the particular retreat context of the *Exercises* but can be seen to also offer guidelines for decision-making in everyday Christian life.[57]

The starting point of the personal transformation process, as Rahner explains, is that during the first week of the retreat, participants are led to become mistrustful of their former lives,[58] which is in accordance with a main principle of the psychology of conceptual change discussed in Chapter 2, namely that an effective motivational intervention often requires some degree of initial "rocking the boat." Regarding how the initial urge to change can be followed up, Ignatius offers three archetypical Election scenarios,[59] which are usually referred to as the *three methods of discernment*. Their significance lies in the fact that they are seen by many as the most authentic generalisable framework for perceiving God's call on one's life. Let us examine the three options one by one.

---

51 E.g. Rahner (*Spiritual Exercises*, 15) submits that "A personal election is the most important thing in an Ignatian retreat."
52 See e.g. Robert, "Union with God," 100, for a detailed discussion.
53 *Spiritual Exercises*, 184.
54 Rahner, *Spiritual Exercises*, 127.
55 Robert, "Union with God," 106.
56 Rahner, *Spiritual Exercises*, 126.
57 See e.g. Lonsdale, *Eyes to See*, 103.
58 Rahner, *Spiritual Exercises*, 126.
59 *Spiritual Exercises*, 175–187.

The first method of discernment involves the Holy Spirit giving someone a direct and specific prompt to follow. This is by definition a *primary visionary message* from God, and as such, it does not have to be accompanied by the experience of consolation; it is, in Christina Astorga's words, "deep and unshakeable,"[60] and Ignatius offers the example of the Apostle Paul's decision to follow the Lord. Such a direct approach will be familiar to contemporary believers attending charismatic churches, where prophecies, words of knowledge and various spiritually received pictures are usually taken very seriously.

The second method of discernment is based on analysing internal emotional movements, that is, reflecting on the consolation and desolation that one experiences (as discussed earlier) and then making a choice along the consolation trajectory, which is accompanied by great joy, hope and peace.[61] In this case, therefore, people rely on the perception of their own emotional states and impulses as indicators of their spiritual alignment with God's purposes. Sparough, Manney and Hipskind emphasise that it is normal to experience a deep unrest in one's heart during this phase: "When the matter is an important one, it stands to reason that the struggle in our conflicted hearts would intensify."[62]

The third method of discernment involves situations when no explicit divine message has been discerned and when there are no salient emotional movements in the person to rely on as an innate compass. In such cases, Ignatius offers two alternatives. First, one may consider rationally all the available options – and thus engage in a form of cost-benefit calculation – in order to weigh and evaluate the advantages, disadvantages and consequences of a possible decision: "Then I must come to a decision in the matter under deliberation because of weightier motives presented to my reason, and not because of any sensual inclination."[63] Alternatively, one may add to this rational evaluation process the power of mental imagery; Ignatius suggests three possible ways to do so:

- "I should represent to myself a man whom I have never seen or known, and whom I would like to see practice all perfection. Then I should consider what I would tell him to do and choose for the greater glory of God our Lord and the greater perfection of his soul."[64]
- "This is to consider what procedure and norm of action I would wish to have followed in making the present choice if I were at the moment of death."[65]

---

60 Astorga, "Ignatian Discernment," 96.
61 Ibid.
62 Sparough, Manney and Hipskind, *What's Your Destiny?* 115.
63 *Spiritual Exercises*, 182.
64 Ibid., 185.
65 Ibid., 186.

- "Let me picture and consider myself as standing in the presence of my judge on the last day, and reflect what decision in the present matter I would then wish to have made."[66]

Regardless of the specific technique applied in the third method of discernment, the final choice needs to be offered to God in prayer so that "the Divine Majesty may deign to accept and confirm it if it is for His greater service and praise."[67] And thus, as Robert concludes, "The union with God experienced in the Election opens out onto the future."[68]

While this discussion of the various approaches may have presented them as distinct options, in reality some aspects of all three will often play a role in arriving at a final decision. Astorga argues this point convincingly when she presents an integrated framework of spiritual discernment.[69] She describes Ignatius's third mode as the preliminary stage that involves gathering facts and pieces of evidence, thinking through the pros and cons, using both reason and mental imagery. Then, in the second mode, one brings the shortlisted options before God in prayer and discerns the movements of consolation or desolation in one's emotional response. Astorga cautions that one should be mindful at this stage "of the deceptions that one can fall into, especially pseudo-consolations and the disguises of evil in what is apparently good,"[70] as well as of the "impulses that come from one's own disordered inclination – timidity, pride, fear, anxiety, anger, ambition, or resentment."[71] Finally, although the first mode of discernment concerns God's sovereign gift when a person is given "a certitude that comes like a light . . . and then one possesses an absolute clarity of one's choice,"[72] several commentators emphasise that even such a direct message may not necessarily be inspired purely by God and needs therefore to be submitted to the other two forms of discernment.[73]

Imaginative prayer

Imaginative (or contemplative) prayer involves the kind of imagery-based approach that the *Meditations on the Life of Christ* and Ignatius's *Spiritual Exercises* have promoted, that is, stepping into a particular scene described in the gospel story and adopting an imaginary eyewitness perspective that can potentially lead to communicating with some of the biblical characters

---

66 Ibid., 187.
67 Ibid., 183.
68 Robert, "Union with God," 110.
69 Astorga, "Ignatian Discernment," 98–99.
70 Ibid., 99.
71 Ibid.
72 Ibid.
73 See e.g. Ivens, *Understanding the Spiritual Exercises*, 136.

in the scene. As we have seen earlier, in Ignatian spirituality this contampla-tive method has been integrated into the fabric of the overall retreat mate-rial, and it is used in combination with other types of prayer in order to create the spiritual context for the retreatant to make a mature decision to transform one's life in harmony with God's purposes. The reason for revisiting this practice in the current section is that the use of the faculty of vision during prayer does not have to be part of such a structured retreat agenda but can also be employed simply to enrich one's everyday prayer life. This point has been powerfully made by Gregory Boyd in his book *See-ing Is Believing: Experience Jesus through Imaginative Prayer*. He begins by pointing out that his personal observation over 25 years of practice has led him to realise that the key to having a rewarding prayer life is to engage one's imagination in a visual manner:

> people who are passionate about prayer tend to be people who, usually without knowing it, use their imaginations in prayer in a way that other people do not. They may "picture" Jesus in their minds when they talk to him. They may "hear" Jesus responding to their words when they pray. They may "see" with the "mind's eye" the person they're praying for and perhaps imaginatively signify that the person being prayed for is benefiting from the prayer. The particulars vary greatly, but in all cases these people vividly and concretely enter into an imaginative world that they experience as real.[74]

The reason why vision can bring such vitality to prayer is related to the capacity of mental imagery to behold an alternative reality in a life-like manner (discussed in Chapter 1). As Boyd emphasises, "seeing is believing," and therefore through seeing in the mind's eye the believer can get immersed in transcendent reality. The main benefit of bringing our human capacity of imagination and mental imagery to prayer is not merely the intensifica-tion of one's prayer life but also the prospect of being able to move beyond what Boyd calls a mere "intellectual Christianity." This, according to Boyd, is ineffective in countering the very sensual deceits of the world, the flesh and the devil surrounding Christians; as he argues, "If our faith is going to be powerful and transformative, it is going to have to be imaginative and experiential."[75] This approach shares a great deal in common with Igna-tian spirituality, because Ignatius also states at the beginning of the *Spir-itual Exercises* that "it is not much knowledge that fills and satisfies the soul, but the intimate understanding and relish of the truth."[76] As already mentioned, Boyd acknowledges this spiritual connection to Ignatian spir-ituality by recognising Ignatius as the person who has "most profoundly

74 Boyd, *Seeing Is Believing*, 15.
75 Ibid., 79.
76 *Spiritual Exercises*, 2.

thought through the role of imagination in prayer,"[77] and in the same way as Ignatius, he, too, calls for Christians to use their faculty of vision in prayer to further their spiritual growth. He has not been alone in this. John English for example states,

> It is good to remember that contemplative prayer has lasted through the Christian centuries. The faith of the church still calls us to contemplation. My confidence in this type of prayer stems more from the fact that holy people in the church have been using it for two thousand years than from the fact that theologians can give me an explanation of it.[78]

Thus, while it is true that the use of mental imagery in Christian practice has been riddled with questions, issues and sometimes with controversies, we have also seen in this chapter that imaginative prayer falls in line with a long tradition of Spirit-filled contemplation in Christianity. We saw in Chapter 5 that just like with other methods of exercising one's faith, care needs to be taken not to abuse the use of vision, but if practiced wisely, imaginative prayer can be seen as a powerful tool whose potential benefits to Christian life cut across denominational boundaries. The enriching value inherent to spirited contemplation has been expressively described by William of St. Thierry as early as the 12th century as follows:

> When we begin not only to understand, but in some way also to touch with our hands and to feel the inner sense of the scriptures, and the power of God's mysteries and sacraments, then Wisdom begins to offer her riches. This touching and feeling is produced by the inner senses when these are well practiced in the art of reading the soul's secrets and the hidden action of God's grace.[79]

When Joshua inherited the leadership of the Israelites from Moses, God's initial instructions to him included the command, "This book of the law shall not depart out of your mouth; you shall meditate on it day and night, so that you may be careful to act in accordance with all that is written in it" (Josh 1:8); the initial verses of the very first Psalm underline the same point:

> Happy are those
>   who do not follow the advice of the wicked,
> or take the path that sinners tread,
>   or sit in the seat of scoffers;
> but their delight is in the law of the LORD,
>   and on his law they meditate day and night.
>   (Ps 1:1–2)

---

77 Boyd, *Seeing Is Believing*, 92.
78 English, *Spiritual Freedom*, 137–138.
79 Cited in Dailey, "The Body and Its Senses," 268.

It is difficult to imagine how meditating on the Scriptures "day and night" could happen without engaging in some form of imaginative prayer; we should also note that such an engagement is described by the Psalmist as leading to happiness and delight, or, using Ignatius's term, to consolation. In our current age, Boyd has observed that people who are able to pursue imaginative prayer experience it as "important, meaningful, and rewarding," and concludes accordingly, "Anyone who experienced what they experience when they pray certainly would do more of it! And anyone who experienced prayer as sheer obligation, as most of us do, would tend to do less of it."[80]

Vision-led Christian leadership and ministry

The primary difference between cultivated vision and the second major theme of this chapter, the application of vision in church leadership and in other Christian ministries, is fundamentally an individual–collective contrast: the practice of cultivated vision focuses on the believers' internal spiritual development whereas the emphasis in leaders' vision is more on how vision can be utilised for serving others more effectively, that is, how it can help believers in their various ministry functions. The conception of the notion of "vision" in the current discussion will be similar to that used in the business world (Chapter 2), referring to an extended, panoramic concept of an ideal future state[81] that exerts considerable motivational power both in leaders and church members as they try to approach the envisaged goals.[82] Yet, we need to reiterate here that even a lavish vision statement in the business world has its initial seed in a leader's personal imagery and private revelation; it is this seed that is then grown into an extended, corporate vision for the whole organisation.[83] Rick Warren captures this point well: "Nothing starts happening until somebody starts dreaming. Every accomplishment started off first as an idea in somebody's mind. It started off as a dream. It started off as a vision. . . ."[84]

---

80 Boyd, *Seeing Is Believing*, 15.
81 In Kouzes and Posner's (*The Leadership Challenge*, 97) words, "an ideal and unique image of the future."
82 The analogy between the usages in business and Christian contexts is well illustrated, for example, by Malphurs and Penfold (*Re:Vision*, 146) when they quote Haddon Robinson: "As Christian leaders we have something in common with Walt Disney. Soon after the completion of Disney World someone said, 'Isn't it too bad that Walt Disney didn't live to see this!' Mike Vance, creative director of Disney Studios, replied, 'He did see it – that's why it's here.'"
83 E.g. Hunter ("Clearing Your Vision," 43) underlines the fact that "in twenty years of ministry I had never seen a committee receive a vision. Committees had offered wonderful methods to accomplish a vision or reach a goal. They had confirmed and refined an individual's insights. But I had never seen vision originate in group process – not in the Bible, not in the church."
84 Warren, "3 Aspects of Vision."

Much of the material in this section will be based on the contemporary literature on vision in Christian leadership and church growth, which shows a strong overlap with business management approaches (to the extent that some of the main authors such as Maxwell, Kouzes and Posner have contributed to both domains). Yet, Christian leaders following a vision-oriented approach are at pains to emphasise that their mode of operation is divinely inspired and has definite biblical analogies.[85] They would argue that the vision they talk about involves a call to fulfil the future hope that God reveals through the "eyes of the heart" of the believer, in accordance with the prayer at the beginning of Ephesians (already cited):

> I pray that the God of our Lord Jesus Christ, the Father of glory, may give you a spirit of wisdom and *revelation* as you come to know him, so that, *with the eyes of your heart enlightened*, you may know what is the hope to which he has called you. . . .
>
> (1:17–18; emphasis added)

In agreement with this assertion, it will set the right tone for the following discussion if we begin with considering how some prominent biblical figures shared features of the visionary leader.

Visionary leaders in the Bible

John Stott offers the following definition of the broad conception of vision that is used in leadership contexts:

> So what is vision? It is an act of seeing, of course, an imaginative perception of things, combining insight and foresight. But more particularly, in the sense in which I am using the word, it is compounded of a deep dissatisfaction with what is and a clear grasp of what could be. It begins with indignation over the status quo, and it grows into the earnest quest for an alternative.[86]

Read this description together with Myles Munroe's definition – "To have vision means to see something coming into view as if it were already there"[87] – and we have a common denominator between diverse biblical leaders such as Moses, King Josiah, Nehemiah and Paul. They all had a longing for a better reality, they all received a divine vision about an alternative future and they all responded to God's visionary call by sharing the

---

85 E.g. Barna (*Power of Vision*, 5) makes this point very clearly: "Vision for ministry is a clear mental image of a preferable future imparted by God to His chosen servants and is based on an accurate understanding of God, self and circumstances."

86 Stott, *Issues Facing Christians*, 487.

87 Munroe, *Principles and Power of Vision*, 45.

foretaste of the brighter future with others, thereby urging them to align themselves with God's purposes. Let us consider briefly the vision of each of these four leaders.

Moses

When God instructed Moses to bring the Israelites out of Egypt (Exod 3:7–10), he did not only give him a command but also a vision of the move from slavery in Egypt "to a good and broad land, a land flowing with milk and honey" (Exod 3:8). It was argued in Chapter 4 that his picturesque description served as powerful guided imagery to energise people and to fill them with hope. Aubrey Malphurs points out that in Moses's case the Bible uniquely describes both how he originally received the divine vision in Exodus 3:7–12 and then how he cast this vision to his people, for example in Deuteronomy 8:7–10.[88] His vision statement presents a sharp contrast between the present and the future:[89]

> For the land that you are about to enter to occupy is not like the land of Egypt, from which you have come, where you sow your seed and irrigate by foot like a vegetable garden. But the land that you are crossing over to occupy is a land of hills and valleys, watered by rain from the sky, a land that the Lord your God looks after.
>
> (Deut 11:10–12)

This vision played a vital role in keeping both Moses and the Israelites going over the years, and as a special reward to Moses, God allowed him to behold the vision also through his physical eyes before he died (Deut 32:48–52).

King Josiah

Josiah was an extraordinary ruler of Judah: "Before him there was no king like him, who turned to the Lord with all his heart, with all his soul, and with all his might, according to all the law of Moses; nor did any like him arise after him" (2 Kgs 23:25). He was comparable to King David – "walked in all the way of his father David" (2 Kgs 22:2) – and in fact, John Goldingay argues that he even "out-Davids David, because 'he did not turn off, right or left' – which could not be said of David."[90] The specific verse of

---

88 Malphurs, *Developing a Vision*, 118.
89 As Brueggemann (*Prophetic Imagination*, 9, 14) sums up, "The alternative consciousness wrought through Moses is characterized by criticizing and energizing. . . . Moses and this narrative create the sense of new realities that can be trusted and relied upon just when the old realities had left us hopeless, it is the task of the prophet to bring to expression the new realities against the more visible ones of the old order."
90 Goldingay, *Old Testament Theology*, 667.

Scripture that Goldingay cites about Josiah – "he did not turn aside to the right or to the left" (2 Kgs 22:2) – also appears in several other places in the Old Testament,[91] referring to observing laws and commands resolutely,[92] and the vision-driven determination underlying the expression is expressed elaborately in Proverbs 4:25–27:

> Let your eyes look directly forward,
>   and your gaze be straight before you.
> Keep straight the path of your feet,
>   and all your ways will be sure.
> Do not swerve[93] to the right or to the left;
>   turn your foot away from evil.

Josiah's vision was of a purified Judah and Jerusalem, purged of any pagan altars, high places, shrines, idols and relics (even dead pagan priests' bones). He accomplished this zealously, even going beyond the borders of Judea (e.g. to Bethel), and he also had the Temple cleansed and repaired. He instituted radical reforms in the religious practices of his time and a particularly remarkable element in his story is that during the restoration of the Temple a copy of the "book of the law" was found (2 Kings 22:8–9), possibly the Pentateuch or some part of it.[94] Reading the book further increased Josiah's zeal and he organised a public reading of it in the Temple for the whole population (23:1–3). As a result, together they made a covenant before the Lord "to follow the Lord, keeping his commandments, his decrees, and his statutes, with all his heart and all his soul, to perform the words of this covenant that were written in this book" (v. 3). In other words, Josiah's vision led him to the discovery of the written report of Moses's earlier vision, which not only inspired him further but also directed him to cast vision to the people by sharing with them the recovered vision report and urging them to transform their lives. His mission was successful and "All the people joined in the covenant" (v. 3).

Nehemiah

Nehemiah's vision of rebuilding the walls of Jerusalem is usually regarded as the textbook illustration of how a divine vision can be received and effectively acted upon. As Malphurs and Penfold underline, the successfully realised initial vision that God put in Nehemiah's heart (Neh 2:12) has grown

---

91 Deut 5:32; 17:11, 20; 28:14; Josh 1:7; 23:6; Prov 4:27.
92 According to Goldingay (ibid., 667), the phrase suggests "the resolute, unwavering, fanatical pursuit of a goal, like that of an athlete running a marathon."
93 Same verb (*nṭh*) used as in the phrase in 2 Kgs 22:2 and the other examples cited.
94 See e.g. Schutz, "Josiah," 1139.

into "a movement of spiritual restoration of repatriated Israel,"[95] which was something much larger than Nehemiah originally expected. A unique feature of Nehemiah's story is that it contains no overt miracles or divine interventions – God's will is fulfilled purely by means of a vision.[96] The Old Testament provides a wealth of details about the process of executing this vision as it devotes an entire book of the Bible to it that draws to a large extent on a first-person account by Nehemiah himself and which is, accordingly, named after him.[97] The next two chapters will cite several aspects of Nehemiah's story to illustrate various vision-related points; from our current perspective, particularly the following five stages of the unfolding story of the realisation of Nehemiah's visionary experience are of special significance:

(a) After hearing some troubling news about the dire state of Jerusalem, Nehemiah, the cupbearer of the Persian King (and thus part of his inner circle), comes to feel a burden ("I sat down and wept, and mourned for days"; 1:4), which often is an initial birth pain of a vision.[98]

(b) Over a period of "fasting and praying before the God of heaven" (1:4) he develops a mature vision of action to "rebuild the wall of Jerusalem" (2:17) so that the Jews who returned from captivity "may no longer suffer disgrace" (v. 17).

(c) Four months after hearing the initial news about Jerusalem, an opportunity finally opens for Nehemiah to step out in faith despite considerable risk ("Then I was very much afraid"; 2:2)[99] and initiate the fulfilment of the vision by putting his case to the king of Persia. His request is met with the king's favour ("the king granted me what I asked, for the gracious hand of my God was upon me"; 2:8) and he is appointed the governor of Judah.

(d) On his arrival to Jerusalem, he casts vision to the local people in order to generate corporate commitment to it, and then models the vision through his own behaviour.

95 Malphurs and Penfold, *Re:Vision*, 43.
96 As Maxwell and Elmore (*Maxwell Leadership Bible*, 590) point out, "no overt miracles occur in the book. Nobody is healed or raised from the dead. God simply answers prayer by providing a leader with favour, strength, and wisdom. Then the work of God is fleshed out in the day-to-day grind of committed workers under one man's gifted leadership – ordinary people enjoying God's blessing as they follow a gifted leader."
97 For a summary of the "Nehemiah Memoir," see e.g. Williamson, *Ezra, Nehemiah*, xxiv-xxviii.
98 Stanley, *Visioneering*, 19.
99 The particular challenge Nehemiah faced concerned the fact that according to Ezra's witness (4:21), the building work in Jerusalem had been suspended earlier in compliance with Artaxerxes' own decree, and therefore Nehemiah was, in effect, intending to petition the king to change his own decree; see e.g. Allen and Laniak, *Ezra, Nehemiah, Esther*, 93; Myers, *Ezra, Nehemiah*, 99.

(e) He pursues the vision by persisting in the face of formidable difficulties and resistance, never failing to believe that "The God of heaven is the one who will give us success" (Neh 2:20).

Thus, the Book of Nehemiah can be seen to offer a comprehensive, stepwise biblical template for the realisation of a divine vision, and it also includes a great deal of trouble-shooting advice.

Paul

Paul's specific visionary experiences have already been addressed in several places in this book, but our current focus is on his overarching vision that the individual experiences amounted to. It all started with the vision of Jesus on the road to Damascus, in which Jesus told Paul, "I have appeared to you for this purpose, to appoint you to serve and testify to the things in which you have seen me and to those in which I will appear to you" (Acts 26:16). Paul describes the ensuing visionary drive in his epistle to the Philippians:

> Not that I have already obtained this or have already reached the goal; but I press on to make it my own, because Christ Jesus has made me his own. Beloved, I do not consider that I have made it my own; but this one thing I do: forgetting what lies behind and straining forward to what lies ahead, I press on toward the goal for the prize of the heavenly call of God in Christ Jesus.
>
> (3:12–14)

In their commentary on this passage, Hawthorne and Martin rightly conclude that "Paul is obsessed with Christ. Nothing else matters but Christ."[100] We should note, however, that the text also adds something more specific: Paul's obsession is with Christ's "*call*" and the "*prize*" that lies ahead. There has been no agreement amongst scholars on what exactly the words "call" and "prize" refer to in the passage, with suggestions ranging from understanding these within an overall sport imagery or in a more abstract way, indicating salvation and a call to be with Christ in heaven.[101] From our vision-specific perspective, it makes sense to equate "the heavenly call of God in Christ Jesus" with the vision Paul received, a reading which is fully consistent with Paul's statement in Galatians: "But when God, who . . . *called* me through his grace, was pleased to *reveal* his Son to me, so that I might proclaim him among the Gentiles" (1:15; emphasis added). Thus, Paul is caught up in a motivational drive fueled and directed by his vision,

---

100 Hawthorne and Martin, *Philippians*, 204.
101 See e.g. Brown, *Philippians*; Fowl, *Philippians*, 162; Hawthorne and Martin, *Philippians*, 210–211.

which is not unlike a "motivational current" documented in motivational psychology with regard to absorbing projects.[102] The prize in such currents is the joy of getting to the envisaged end and experiencing the desired vision, and the Philippians passage does indeed highlight the "pressing on toward the goal for the prize of the heavenly call."

Vision-led motivational currents are powerful energy surges, and Paul talks about the binding strength of his vision in several places. For example, in 1 Corinthians 9:16 he states, "for an obligation is laid on me, and woe to me if I do not proclaim the gospel!" and Bill Hybels paraphrases Paul's declarations in Acts 20:24 ("But I do not count my life of any value to myself, if only I may finish my course and the ministry that I received from the Lord Jesus") as follows: "The moment I received my vision from God, fulfilling that vision became the pressing priority of my life."[103] Thus, these considerations underpin Malphurs and Penfold's conclusion that "The apostle Paul, perhaps better than any other human in the New Testament, defines the character of vision-driven leadership."[104]

Vision in contemporary Christian ministry

The use of the term "vision" in contemporary church contexts in the meaning of an ideal future scenario is a relatively new phenomenon. It was originally borrowed from the business world, where "vision" started to appear in the 1980s and then, as George Barna explains, "without warning, vision became the hottest topic around."[105] We saw in Chapter 2 the influential role played in this respect by Kouzes and Posner's bestselling title, *The Leadership Challenge*,[106] whose first edition was published in 1987, and in 2004 the same authors edited an anthology on *Christian Reflections on the Leadership Challenge*,[107] for which they invited a stellar group of Christian contributors (including John Maxwell, Ken Blanchard and Nancy Ortberg) to reflect on the Christian relevance of the five key principles of the original book. In this volume, the president of Wesley Theological Seminary (Washington, DC), David McAllister-Wilson, recounts how in the 1990s he started to read books on secular leadership (including the first edition of *The Leadership Challenge*) in order to find transferable concepts that could be utilised to help students to become effective church leaders and thus to re-vitalise the declining "Mainline Protestantism."[108]

---

102 See Dörnyei et al., *Motivational Currents*.
103 Hybels, *Courageous Leadership*, 36.
104 Malphurs and Penfold, *Re:Vision*, 45.
105 Barna, *Power of Vision*, 9.
106 Kouzes and Posner, *The Leadership Challenge*.
107 Kouzes and Posner, *Christian Reflections*.
108 McAllister-Wilson, "Shared Vision," 55.

The term "vision" was an obvious candidate to adopt from the market-place for Christian contexts, partly because, as Malphurs remembers, it was seen as "a good biblical concept,"[109] and partly because although the business literature was aimed at secular audiences, many of the works (including *The Leadership Challenge*) were written by Christian authors and were compatible with a Christian ethos. The term rapidly took root because of the shared belief in Christian leadership circles that "Vision isn't everything, but it's the beginning of everything,"[110] and Proverbs 29:18 – "where there is no vision, the people perish" (KJV)[111] – has become an oft-cited unofficial slogan of the new approach. There is no doubt that the current zeitgeist promotes vision-led leadership in some church circles;[112] for example, T. D. Jakes states that "When I talk with young pastors today, most of them tell me they assumed they were starting a church that needed to function like a successful business."[113] Having said that, we also need to recognise that there is a fundamental difference between notions of vision in the world of business and in church leadership, as the former concerns *human* aspirations while the latter *divine* vision, that is, God's purposes for humans. Let us examine the consequences of this disparity.

Human vision and God's vision for humans

In a seminal paper on "Building Your Company's Vision," published in the *Harvard Business Review*, James Collin and Jerry Porras argue that "It makes no sense to analyse whether an envisioned future is the right one. With a creation – and the task is creation of a future, not prediction – there can be no right answer."[114] What matters instead, according to these authors, is that the envisioned future should be "so exciting in its own right that it would continue to keep the organization motivated even if the leaders who set the goal disappeared."[115] In other words, vision in the business sense is evaluated not on the basis of whether it is right or wrong, but rather solely on the basis of *how* it does the job, that is, how effective it is in

---

109 Malphurs, *Developing a Vision*, 14.
110 McAllister-Wilson, "Shared Vision," 56.
111 Although this proverb is typically quoted using the translation of the King James Version, more modern translations tend to suggest "cast off restrain" instead of "perish," which is less dramatic but still retains the negative connotation. Bill Johnson (*Supernatural Power*, 66) submits that a more accurate and complete translation would be: "Without a prophetic revelation, the people go unrestrained, walking in circles, having no certain destiny."
112 Much of the vision-specific literature has been written by leaders of non-denominational Protestant (mega)churches mostly but not exclusively in North America.
113 Jakes, *Build Your Vision*, 46.
114 Collins and Porras, "Company Vision," 75.
115 Ibid.

giving an organisation direction and energy. This is, however, the very point where secular and divine visions depart, because as Barna succinctly summarises, "While books by Sculley [former CEO of Pepsi and Apple] and other authors underscore the importance of vision in the business world, they fail to include an irreplaceable factor in the equation from a Christian perspective: the mind of God."[116] An effective vision in the corporate world concerns a good human idea about the future to which the leaders' imagination adds vivid details, thereby enabling the envisaged reality to emerge and impact the whole organisation. In contrast, an effective vision in the Christian world concerns a *divine* idea which is discerned by the recipient through his/her faculty of internal senses, thereby enabling believers to carry out God's purposes when the time is right. Andy Stanley sums up this distinction expressively:

> We have all read something about goal setting. If you believe – you can achieve! You know the drill. But here is where we part ways with the secular motivational gurus of our culture. The average person has the right to dream his own dreams and develop his own picture of what his future could and should be. But at the cross, those of us who have sworn allegiance to the Saviour lost that right. After all, we are not our own.[117]

Does God have a specific plan for everybody?

Thus, in contrast to vision in business, Christian vision is understood as a means to get aligned with God's purposes rather than to realise one's own aspirations; as Myles Munroe explicitly stated, "Vision isn't about us. It's about God and His purposes."[118] This and similar statements made by contemporary Christian leadership experts rest on the belief that God has a concrete plan for every human being that can be discerned through the visionary channel.[119] Is there any concrete biblical warrant for this belief? Arguably the most often cited verse of Scripture to support this claim has been Ephesians 2:10: "For we are God's workmanship, created in Christ Jesus to do good works, which God prepared in advance for us to do." However, commentators have been divided about how specific the preconceived divine plans are that the verse implies. For example, Pheme Perkins infers from this verse that "Every Christian has some 'good works' that are his or her divine calling,"[120] while Francis Foulkes states, "This does not of

116 Barna, *Power of Vision*, 60.
117 Stanley, *Visioneering*, 12–13.
118 Munroe, *Principles and Power of Vision*, 61.
119 E.g. "God has placed His eternal purpose in your heart" (Munroe, ibid., 61); "God has a vision for your life" (Stanley, *Visioneering*, 14).
120 Perkins, *Letter to the Ephesians*, 394–395; for a similar take, see e.g. Thielman, *Ephesians*, 146; Bratcher and Nida, *Ephesians*, 48.

necessity mean that there are particular good works that are God's purpose for us. . . . probably it is rather the whole course of life that is on view here."[121] This uncertainty in interpretation warrants further examination of the issue.

An inspection of the biblical corpus suggests that there may not be any incontestable declarations in the Bible that state unequivocally that God has a concrete plan for every single believer. Besides Ephesians 2:10, the verse that comes closest to this target is possibly Psalm 57:2 – "I cry to God Most High, to God who fulfils his purpose for me" – but as this was a psalm attributed to King David, the first person singular might be read that God only had a special plan for him as Israel's king. We do find in the Scriptures, however, a number of verses that, taken together, do support the existence of a divine purpose for individual believers. To start with, Hebrews 13:21 highlights the importance of God's will in human conduct – "May the God of peace . . . equip you with everything good for doing his will, and may he work in us what is pleasing to him" – and Proverbs 20:24 asserts that "A man's steps are directed by the LORD. How then can anyone understand his own way?" The importance of divine agency is also underlined in Jeremiah 10:23 – "I know, O Lord, that the way of human beings is not in their control, that mortals as they walk cannot direct their steps" – and two other proverbs emphasise the futility of human plans if they are not aligned with those of God: "Many are the plans in a man's heart, but it is the LORD'S purpose that prevails" (19:21) and "In his heart a man plans his course, but the LORD determines his steps" (16:9). This point is made most explicitly in Psalm 127:1 – "Unless the Lord builds the house, those who build it labour in vain" – and a similar message is offered in Lamentations 3:37: "Who can speak and have it happen if the Lord has not decreed it?" Finally, Psalm 37:23 reiterates this point in an affirmative manner: "Our steps are made firm by the Lord, when he delights in our way."

In sum, a consistent message emerges in the Scriptures that places God's vision for humans *over* human vision and which urges people to trust the Lord and he will act. This is the central idea in the oft-quoted passage, "Trust in the LORD with all your heart and lean not on your own understanding; in all your ways acknowledge him, and he will make your paths straight" (Prov 3:5–6), and the point could not have been made any more explicit in Psalm 37:5: "Commit your way to the LORD; trust in him, and he will act," also reiterated in Proverbs: "Commit your work to the Lord, and your plans will be established" (16:3). Taking the various biblical teachings and admonitions cited together, the overall picture is one that places the believers' dependence on God with all their plans and actions on top of everything, and such a recurring emphasis simply would not make sense if God did not have something in store for every believer to depend on. Without

---

121 Foulkes, *Ephesians*, 85; for a similar take, see e.g. Klein, "Ephesians," 71.

wanting to sound frivolous, when the Scriptures foreground the significance of "God ideas" over "good ideas" (to take an expressive contrast frequently mentioned in the church leadership literature[122]), this indicates that the former do exist.

We should also note, however, what is *not* said in any of these messages, namely that human initiatives, ideas and contributions are *not* required. The cited passages suggest that human schemes become pointless only if they are in discord with God's purposes and directions. Indeed, one *needs* to take steps for God to be able to direct those steps (Prov 16:9), and steps are also *needed* so that God can make them firm (Ps 37:23); similarly, people *need* to get involved in planning so that God can establish their plans (Prov 16:3). It appears therefore that the Scriptures promote a synthesis of human and divine agency, with the former only bearing fruit if it is aligned with the latter. This also appears to be the main message of Jesus' teaching in John 15:5: "I am the vine; you are the branches. If you remain in me and I in you, you will bear much fruit; apart from me you can do nothing."

The last two chapters of this book will explore how an alignment with God's purposes can be achieved in practical terms, but in order to create a solid foundation for that discussion, it is important to elucidate here a distinctive characteristic of vision in Christian life and ministry, namely that the alignment between divine vision and human behaviour can occur at three separate although interrelated levels: at the *leadership level*, at the *collective organisation level* and at the *individual believer's level*. It stands to reason that in order for vision to release the full extent of its transformational potential, the three levels need to interact with each other in a harmonious manner, so let us conclude this chapter by examining the three levels of vision and how they can complement each other.

Leadership vision, collective vision and individual vision

The contemporary Christian literature on vision has shown a certain amount of ambiguity in stipulating its target audience, sometimes aiming specifically at church leaders, at other times speaking to believers in general. One can sympathise with the authors' dilemma: on the one hand, within church contexts a leader is arguably in the best position to realise God's vision for the whole congregation, and church leaders are also the closest parallels to business leaders when authors import various lessons from the business world on how to run a church; on the other hand, we have also seen that even broad visions impacting whole organisations and ministries have their roots in individual visionary experiences. We need also to remember that the recipients of such visions may not actually be in a leadership role at the time

---

122 E.g. Lovejoy (*Vision*, 26) states, "There's a big difference between a good idea and a God idea. . . . Vision is something revealed by God"; see also Stanley, *Visioneering*, 25.

they first discern God's message, as it may be the vision itself that catapults them into a position of influence. Two other considerations further blur the picture:

- Congregational churches and non-denominational congregations are typically led by *leadership teams* that sometimes consist of several layers, and therefore even visionary content relevant to "church leaders" may actually concern a wider segment of church membership.[123]
- Not all individual visions may find their best outworking in a church framework; some may concern Christian para-church ministries (e.g. in the areas of missionary outreach, social action or healing and deliverance), while others may simply offer guidelines for believers' everyday Christian walk/service without pointing them towards any sort of leadership position.

Thus, it is virtually impossible to draw the line between vision's different spheres of relevance for service, which is in fact consistent with Paul's teaching that the body of Christ comprises many different members with their unique roles and gifting, all of whose joint service is needed for the healthy functioning of the church (Rom 12:4–8; see also Eph 4:11–16). Interestingly, in most cases the lack of a firm specification of the layer of vision does not seem to affect the overall discussion adversely: because vision is related to a general human faculty, much of the material on vision in Christian life is sufficiently generic to apply to both members and leaders of a church, while also being relevant to the pursuit of a wide range of Christian ministries. Accordingly, an inclusive approach is quite common in the contemporary vision literature in this respect, as illustrated for example by the subtitle of Myles Munroe's book on vision: *Discover and Apply God's Plan for Your Life and Ministry*.[124] Interestingly, a similarly titled book on vision by George Barna highlights in its subtitle another area of integration, that of the "personal and corporate" levels: *Keys to Achieving Personal and Corporate Destiny*.[125] This foregrounds the third main aspect of vision in Christian life, *collective vision*.

Collective vision

In Chapter 2 we saw that vision in business management involves some form of sharing with a larger constituency for the purpose of furthering the

---

123 E.g. Malphurs (*Developing a Vision*, 60) points out that "In the church the driving wheels are people of influence who are found at different levels of leadership. Some may be on the staff while others are on the church's board(s). Some are involved in other areas of the ministry from teaching a class of adults to serving in the nursery."

124 Barna, *Power of Vision*.

125 Munroe, *Principles and Power of Vision*.

organisation, and the effectiveness of a vision in business is assessed on the basis of how it manages to rally the troops and give the company a collective direction. This characteristic is just as relevant for churches and ministries as for business organisations, as reflected, for example, by the following quotation by Shawn Lovejoy, which concerns church vision but which could have equally come out of a business leaders' manual: "A vision is only as strong as it can be shared and applied. Having a vision is the starting point, not the finish line. Our next leadership task is to pass it on so that others can make it their own."[126] Success in the area of sharing the vision promises ample rewards, because, as Dave Gilpin has found, "If the leader's vision becomes every person's vision, the achievement levels will break all records."[127]

There are several valuable publications that offer advice on how Christian leaders can best communicate and cast vision,[128] but the focus of the current discussion is not so much on such leadership strategies as on the nature of the collective vision itself and how it can emerge from individually experienced mental images. So, how can the personal image of a possible future scenario grow into a collective vision that will be shared by a whole community of believers? Gilpin rightly points out that the common understanding of this process is that it occurs through "vision casting," which is "all about telling people what they'll be up to in five years' time and what projects will have come to pass."[129] There is nothing wrong with this practice and, if delivered appropriately, a well-crafted vision statement can result in a state that, in Bill Hybels's words, "people's hearts are stirred enough to shout, 'Count me in!'"[130] There are several presentation techniques that can increase the effectiveness of casting vision,[131] but when the goal is to enlist others in a God-mandated exercise with potential life-changing consequences, one crucial

---

126 Lovejoy, *Vision*, 63.
127 Gilpin, *Confessions of a Confused Leader*, 67.
128 E.g. Gilpin, ibid; Hybels, *Axiom*; Malphurs, *Developing a Vision*; Maxwell, *Laws of Leadership*; Stanley, *Visioneering*.
129 Gilpin, *Confessions of a Confused Leader*, 13.
130 Hybels, *Axiom*, 31.
131 In summarising how transformational leaders communicate visions in the field of education in a way that those should transcend the individual members' self-interest, Dörnyei and Kubanyiova (*Motivating Learners*, 87–88) list the following strategies, most of which are directly transferrable to church/mission environments:

- articulating the vision precisely, framed within the "big picture" outlining both the desired end state and the proposed route towards it;
- expressing the vision in highly engaging terms and offering a vividly detailed description of a future that people can readily picture, thereby making a compelling case and an inspirational appeal for it;
- displaying infectious enthusiasm in the group/organisation for the project;
- setting high performance expectations in combination with expressing confidence that the goals will be achieved;
- offering encouragement to the group members and instilling pride in them for being associated with the project;

step is indispensable: aligning the members' individual visions with the over-all organisational vision. Kouzes and Posner make this point very clearly:

> Having your vision of the future isn't enough, however. Others must be able to see themselves in that future. You can't impose your vision on others; it has to be something that has meaning to them, not just to you. Leaders enlist others in a common vision by appealing to shared aspirations. . . . There is in all people a deep yearning to make a differ-ence. We want to know that we've done something on this earth, that there's a purpose to our existence. . . . Exemplary Christian leaders are able to release this human longing by communicating the meaning and significance of what people do – whether in the church, the workplace, or the community – so that they understand their own important role in creating it.[132]

In other words, a compelling and lasting collective vision will only emerge if it can accommodate the participants' individual dreams. If church members can envisage themselves accomplishing something as part of pursuing the overall vision of the church that is congruent with their own core values and aspirations, they will be completely sold on the project. McAllister-Wilson underlines the significance of the maxim "People support what they help to create,"[133] thereby echoing Kouzes and Posner's final point in the earlier quote, and Rick Warren's following definition of a healthy church argues along the same line:

> The best kept secret in the Church is that people are dying to make a contribution with their lives. We are made for ministry! When eve-ryone uses their unique, God-given SHAPE to make a difference for Jesus' sake in your community, you'll make a tangible, visible differ-ence in your community. The church that understands this, and con-tinually calls people to a vision where every member can express his or her uniqueness in ministry, will experience amazing vitality, health and growth.[134]

- "walking the talk," that is communicating the vision in both words and deeds, and leading by example;
- aligning fully all the main administrative, financial and personnel decisions within the group with the spirit of the vision;
- emphasising the vision with symbolic actions such as ceremonies to celebrate it and assemblies to honour any effort towards it;
- communicating key aspects of the vision visually in mottos, logos, letterheads, ban-ners, posters, etc.

132 Kouzes and Posner, *Christian Reflections*, 18.
133 McAllister-Wilson, "Shared Vision," 64.
134 Warren, "Restate Your Vision."

In other words, as Warren emphasises, people are looking for significance, and a powerful collective vision conveys to people the sense that they will find significance by partaking in the journey.[135] Ken Blanchard calls the leadership style that is focused on promoting and accommodating other people's visions the "servant leader," and explains that for such leaders "the main reason for leading is to help other people win. Put another way, it's to help people live according to the vision God placed inside them."[136] And according to Max De Pree, the church leader does not even have to be the author of the vision; visions can come from many different sources, and the leader's main responsibility is to be the chief carrier of the vision.[137] Thus, the emergence of a potent collective vision involves an intriguing and subtle process of alignment and blending, not unlike a gradually unfolding dance performed jointly by the visionary, the church leadership and the congregation.[138]

Summary

This chapter has explored two established approaches to applying vision for the purpose of enriching Christian life, namely cultivated vision and vision-led church/ministry leadership. Although both are different from biblical vision proper – that is, from receiving divine messages as described in Chapters 3 and 4 – both are aimed at utilising the human faculty of mental imagery to "get onto the divine wavelength," thereby connecting to transcendent reality. Cultivated vision involves intentionally activating mental imagery by adding visualisation to prayer or the reading of Scripture, with the integrity of the process protected by focusing on Jesus, who is the image of God. By envisaging the earthly ministry of the "Father's only Son," believers hope to have a glimpse of divine glory. As a result, gospel meditation became a popular Christian practice in the late Middle Ages and the best-known "handbook" for offering "holy" guided imagery – *Meditations on the Life of Christ* – became an international bestseller. Drawing on these traditions, St. Ignatius of Loyola developed a coherent vision-based training programme that elevated gospel meditation to a new level of sophistication by embedding it in a programme of spiritual growth and by including several safeguards against subjective or diabolical corruption. The specific relevance of Ignatian spirituality to the current book is that it utilises vision for the explicit purpose of transforming the participants. Five hundred years after its initiation, the principles of Ignatius's vision-led retreats are still

---

135 Warren, "7 Ways to Help."
136 Blanchard, "Encourage the Heart," 104.
137 De Pree, "Visionary Jazz," 28.
138 Stanley (*Visioneering*, 90) states in this respect: "No one accomplishes a God-given vision alone. Whether your vision involves the salvation of a friend or the launching of an organization, it is going to take a team. A team whose imaginations are in alignment."

widely practised within the Jesuit order and beyond, and imaginative prayer has come to be seen as a highly effective method of Spirit-led contemplation.

The harnessing of the motivational qualities of the vision of a better future – which visionary church leaders do – is somewhat different from the principles of cultivated vision. Rather than transporting the individual believer's soul heavenwards with the help of mental imagery, it concerns a collective enterprise through discerning God's plans for serving others more effectively and guiding communities of believers in their various ministry functions. In this sense, this concept of Christian vision shares a lot in common with vision in business leadership, and indeed, many of the influential Christian writers on the subject are also recognised leadership experts in the secular world. Yet, there is a fundamental difference between the notion of vision in the world of business and in church leadership, most notably that the former concerns human aspirations for their own sake while the latter is centred around God's purposes for humans revealed in divine vision. As was argued in this chapter, while there may not be a single verse of Scripture that unequivocally declares that God has a specific plan for everybody, we do find much biblical teaching to the effect that it is God's purposes rather than purely human planning that really matter. This being the case, motivational vision can be understood as a compass for synchronising human plans with divine purpose.

Finally, the chapter addressed a distinctive characteristic of vision in Christian life and ministry, namely that the alignment between divine vision and human behaviour can occur at three separate although interrelated levels: at the *leadership level*, at the *collective organisation level* and at the ind*ividual believer's level*. It was argued that in order to transform church communities, the leaders' individual vision needs to be turned into a shared, collective vision for the whole church community, and a lasting collective vision will only emerge if it can accommodate the participants' individual dreams.

References

Allen, Leslie C., and Timothy S. Laniak. 2003. *Ezra, Nehemiah, Esther*. Understanding the Bible. Grand Rapids, MI: Baker Books.

Aschenbrenner, George A. 2004. *Stretched for Greater Glory: What to Expect from the Spiritual Exercises*. Chicago: Loyola Press.

Astorga, Christina A. 2005. "Ignatian Discernment: A Critical Contemporary Reading for Christian Decision Making." *Horizons* 32, no. 1: 72–99.

Barna, George. 2009. *The Power of Vision: Discover and Apply God's Plan for Your Life and Ministry*. Ventura, CA: Regal.

Behm, Johannes. 1964. "Ἀνάμνησις, Ὑπόμνησις." In *Theological Dictionary of the New Testament*, edited by Gerhard Kittel, Geoffrey. W. Bromiley and Gerhard Friedrich, 348–49. Grand Rapids, MI: Eerdmans.

Blanchard, Ken. 2004. "Reflections on Encourage the Heart." In *Christian Reflections on the Leadership Challenge*, edited by James M. Kouzes and Barry Z. Posner, 101–16. San Francisco: Jossey-Bass.

162 Cultivated vision, vision-led ministry

Boyd, Gregory A. 2004. _Seeing Is Believing: Experience Jesus through Imaginative Prayer_. Grand Rapids, MI: Baker Books.
Bratcher, Robert G., and Eugene Albert Nida. 1982. _A Translator's Handbook on Paul's Letter to the Ephesians_. New York: United Bible Societies.
Brown, Derek R. 2013. _Lexham Bible Guide: Philippians_. Bellingham, WA: Lexham Press.
Brueggemann, Walter. 2001. _The Prophetic Imagination_. 2nd ed. Minneapolis, MN: Fortress.
Collins, James C., and Jerry I. Porras. 1996. "Building Your Company's Vision." _Harvard Business Review_ 74, no. 5: 65–77.
Dailey, Patricia. 2012. "The Body and Its Senses." In _The Cambridge Companion to Christian Mysticism_, edited by Amy Hollywood and Patricia Zoltán Beckman, 264–76. Cambridge: Cambridge University Press.
De Pree, Max. 1997. "Visionary Jazz." In _Renewing Your Church through Vision and Planning: 30 Strategies to Transform Your Ministry_, edited by Marshall Shelley, 27–33. Minneapolis, MN: Bethany House.
Dörnyei, Zoltán, Alastair Henry, and Christine Muir. 2016. _Motivational Currents in Language Learning: Frameworks for Focused Interventions_. New York: Routledge.
Dörnyei, Zoltán, and Maggie Kubanyiova. 2014. _Motivating Learners, Motivating Teachers: Building Vision in the Language Classroom_. Cambridge: Cambridge University Press.
English, John J. 1995. _Spiritual Freedom: From an Experience of the Ignatian Exercises to the Art of Spiritual Guidance_. 2nd ed. Chicago: Loyola University Press.
Ensley, Eddie. 2000. _Visions: The Soul's Path to the Sacred_. Chicago: Loyola Press.
Foulkes, Francis. 1989. _Ephesians_. Tyndale New Testament Commentaries 10. Downers Grove, IL: IVP Academic.
Fowl, Stephen E. 2005. _Philippians_. Grand Rapids, MI: Eerdmans.
Gallagher, Timothy M. 2008. _Meditation and Contemplation: An Ignatian Guide to Praying with Scripture_. New York: Crossroad.
Gilpin, Dave. 2006. _Jesus, Save Me from Your Followers: Confessions of a Confused Leader_. Chichester: New Wine Press.
Goldingay, John. 2003. _Old Testament Theology 1: Israel's Gospel_. Downers Grove, IL: InterVarsity Press.
Green, Thomas H. 2006. _Opening to God: A Guide to Prayer_. Rev. ed. Notre Dame, IN: Ave Maria Press.
Hawthorne, Gerald F., and Ralph P. Martin. 2004. _Philippians_. Word Biblical Commentary 43. Nashville, TN: Thomas Nelson.
Hunter, Joel C. 1997. "Clearing Your Vision." In _Renewing Your Church through Vision and Planning: 30 Strategies to Transform Your Ministry_, edited by Marshall Shelley, 43–49. Minneapolis, MN: Bethany House.
Hybels, Bill. 2002. _Courageous Leadership_. Grand Rapids, MI: Zondervan.
Hybels, Bill. 2008. _Axiom: Powerful Leadership Proverbs_. Grand Rapids, MI: Zondervan.
Ivens, Michael. 1998. _Understanding the Spiritual Exercises: Text and Commentary. A Handbook for Retreat Directors_. Leominster, UK: Gracewing.
Jakes, T. D. 2017. _Soar: Build Your Vision from the Ground Up_. New York: FaithWords.
Johnson, Bill. 2005. _The Supernatural Power of a Transformed Mind: Access to a Life of Miracles_. Shippensburg, PA: Destiny Image.

Karnes, Michelle. 2011. *Imagination, Meditation, and Cognition in the Middle Ages*. Chicago: University of Chicago Press.

Kelly, J. N. D. 1977. *Early Christian Doctrines*. 5th ed. London: A & C Black.

Klein, William W. 2006. "Ephesians." In *The Expositor's Bible Commentary: Ephesians – Philemon (Revised Edition)*, edited by Tremper III Longman and David E. Garland, 19–173. Grand Rapids, MI: Zondervan.

Kouzes, James M., and Barry Z. Posner, eds. 2004. *Christian Reflections on the Leadership Challenge*. San Francisco: Jossey-Bass.

Kouzes, James M., and Barry Z. Posner. 2017. *The Leadership Challenge: How to Make Extraordinary Things Happen in Organisations*. 6th ed. Hoboken, NJ: Wiley.

Lonsdale, David. 2000. *Eyes to See, Ears to Hear: An Introduction to Ignatian Spirituality*. London: Darton, Longman and Todd.

Lovejoy, Shawn. 2016. *Be Mean About the Vision: Preserving and Protecting What Matters*. Nashville, TN: Thomas Nelson.

Malphurs, Aubrey. 2015. *Developing a Vision for Ministry*. 3rd ed. Grand Rapids, MI: Baker Books.

Malphurs, Aubrey, and Gordon E. Penfold. 2014. *Re:Vision: The Key to Transforming Your Church*. Grand Rapids, MI: Baker Books.

Maxwell, John C. 2007. *The 21 Irrefutable Laws of Leadership: Follow Them and People Will Follow You*. Nashville, TN: Thomas Nelson.

Maxwell, John C., and Tim Elmore. 2007. *The Maxwell Leadership Bible*. Nashville, TN: Thomas Nelson.

McAllister-Wilson, David. 2004. "Reflections on Inspire a Shared Vision." In *Christian Reflections on the Leadership Challenge*, edited by James M. Kouzes and Barry Z. Posner, 55–68. San Francisco: Jossey-Bass.

McGinn, Bernard. 2006. *The Essential Writings of Christian Mysticism*. New York: Modern Library.

Munroe, Myles. 2003. *The Principles and Power of Vision: Keys to Achieving Personal and Corporate Destiny*. New Kensington, PA: Whitaker House.

Myers, Jacob M. 1965. *Ezra, Nehemiah*. Anchor Yale Bible 17. New Haven, CT: Yale University Press.

Newman, Barbara. 2005. "What Did It Mean to Say "I Saw"? The Clash between Theory and Practice in Medieval Visionary Culture." *Speculum* 80, no. 1: 1–43.

O'Brien, Kevin. 2011. *The Ignatian Adventure: Experiencing the Spiritual Exercises of Saint Ignatius in Daily Life*. Chicago: Loyola Press.

O'Loughlin, Thomas. 2015. *The Eucharist: Origins and Contemporary Understandings*. London: Bloomsbury T&T Clark.

Perkins, Pheme. 1997. *Ephesians*. Nashville, TN: Abingdon.

Perkins, Pheme. 2000. "The Letter to the Ephesians: Introduction, Commentary, and Reflections." In *The New Interpreter's Bible*, edited by Leander E. Keck, 349–466. Nashville, TN: Abingdon.

Puhl, Louis, J., ed. 1951. *The Spiritual Exercises of St Ignatius: A New Translation Based on Studies in the Language of the Autograph*. Washington, DC: Newman Press.

Ragusa, Isa, and Rosalie B. Green, eds. 1961. *Meditations on the Life of Christ: An Illustrated Manuscript of the Fourteenth Century*. Princeton, NJ: Princeton University Press.

Rahner, Karl. 1967. *Spiritual Exercises*. Translated by Kenneth Baker. London: Sheed and Ward.

Robert, Sylvie. 2002. "Union with God in the Ignatian Election." *Way Supplement* 103: 100–12.

Rowland, Christopher (with Patricia Gibbons, and Vicente Dobroruka). 2006. "Visionary Experience in Ancient Judaism and Christianity." In *Paradise Now: Essays on Early Jewish and Christian Mysticism*, edited by April D. DeConick, 41–56. Atlanta, GA: Society of Biblical Literature.

Sargent, Michael G. 1992. "Introduction." In *Nicholas Love's Mirror of the Blessed Life of Jesus Christ: A Critical Edition Based on Cambridge University Library Additional Mss 6578 and 6686*, edited by Michael G. Sargent, ix–cxlii. New York: Garland.

Sargent, Michael G., ed. 1992. *Nicholas Love's Mirror of the Blessed Life of Jesus Christ: A Critical Edition Based on Cambridge University Library Additional Mss 6578 and 6686*. New York: Garland.

Schutz, S. J. 1988. "Josiah." In *The International Standard Bible Encyclopedia, Revised*, edited by Geoffrey W. Bromiley, 1138–39. Grand Rapids, MI: Eerdmans.

Sparough, Michael J., Jim Manney, and Tim Hipskind. 2010. *What's Your Destiny? How to Make Choices with Confidence and Clarity*. Chicago: Loyola Press.

Spinks, Bryan D. 2013. *Do This in Remembrance of Me: The Eucharist from the Early Church to the Present Day*. London: SCM.

Stanley, Andy. 1999. *Visioneering: God's Blueprint for Developing and Maintaining Vision*. Colorado Springs, CO: Multnomah Books.

Stott, John. 2011. *Issues Facing Christians Today*. 4th ed. Grand Rapids, MI: Zondervan.

Thielman, Frank. 2010. *Ephesians*. Grand Rapids, MI: Baker Academic.

Thiselton, Anthony C. *The Spck Dictionary of Theology and Hermeneutics*. London: SPCK, 2015.

Tóth, Peter, and Dávid Falvay. 2014. "New Light on the Date and Authorship of the Meditationes Vitae Christi." In *Devotional Culture in Late Medieval England and Europe: Diverse Imaginations of Christ's Life*, edited by Stephen Kelly and Ryan Perry, 17–105. Turnhout: Brepols.

Warren, Rick. 2012. "7 Ways to Help Others Understand the Vision." In *Pastors.com*. https://pastors.com/how-to-share-gods-vision-for-your-church/.

Warren, Rick. 2013. "Restate Your Church Vision Every 30 Days." In *Pastors.com*. https://pastors.com/the-nehemiah-principle-vision/.

Warren, Rick. 2017. "3 Aspects of the Vision God Has for Your Church." In *Pastors.com*. https://pastors.com/3-parts-of-vision/.

Williamson, H. G. M. 1985. *Ezra, Nehemiah*. Word Biblical Commentary 16. Dallas, TX: Word Books.

7 Vision in the Christian life I
Discerning God's call

Having surveyed the various understandings and applications of vision in several scholarly disciplines and applied domains, the final part of this book will consider how the lessons drawn from these fields can be utilised for the purpose of enriching Christian life and ministry. The practical nature of this discussion will be best served by organising the material of the current chapter around six questions pertinent to the issue: (1) What does vision involve in a contemporary Christian context? (2) What are the main features of an effective Christian vision? (3) What is vision like for the whole church community? (4) How can we generate a Christian vision? (5) How can we be sure that the vision we have received is from God? (6) How long do we need to wait before starting to implement a vision? The answers will partly draw on the material presented in the earlier chapters and partly on the writings of contemporary Christian leadership experts and visionary leaders[1] whose observations and personal accounts are given authority by the successful realisation of their own visions in real-life settings.

What does vision involve in a contemporary Christian context?

In the previous chapters we have examined three somewhat different aspects of vision – *mental imagery* (in a neuroscientific sense), *divine message* (in a biblical sense) and *ideal future scenario* (in a leadership sense) – and the way in which contemporary Christian vision will be understood in this chapter integrates all these three: (a) it utilises the purposeful deployment of sensory imagination as discussed in psychological theories; (b) it follows the main principle of biblical imagery in that vision will be viewed as the channel of receiving divine guidance; and (c) it adopts the transformational agenda of vision as a desirable future state, that is, "a picture of the future that produces passion."[2]

---

1 E.g. George Barna, Tommy Barnett, Gregory Boyd, Dave Gilpin, Bill Hybels, Shawn Love-joy, Aubrey Malphurs, Gordon Penfold, John Maxwell, Andy Stanley and Rick Warren.
2 Hybels, *Courageous Leadership*, 32.

This integrative approach is not unlike the one that underlies the applications of vision reviewed in Chapter 6, namely cultivated vision and vision in leadership contexts. However, cultivated vision (especially gospel meditation and imaginative prayer) has been less articulate on the motivational direction of applying vision (as the focus is on the experience of resting in Jesus' presence rather than on the fruit of the vision), while visionary leadership has been less concerned with utilising vision for the development/transformation of individuals (rather than organisations). The closest parallel to the present conception of Christian vision has been offered by Ignatian spirituality, which combines the principles of cultivated vision with a programme for transforming individual lives (through the Election). The following discussion adopts a similar agenda and explores, in effect, the question that the rich man asked Jesus in Matthew 19:16: "Teacher, what good deed must I do to have eternal life?" That is, how can believers best serve God in their daily lives?

We should note as a preliminary that viewing Christian vision primarily as part of a gradual process of discerning God's call does not go against more established understandings of perceiving vision, such as prophesying, receiving oracular pictures or words of knowledge and having prophetic dreams or other forms of religious experience with a vision content. The Bible contains several examples when God delivers direct, and even dramatic, messages to certain individuals, as evidenced by the directive to Paul on the road to Damascus, which went against all the convictions of the would-be Apostle, or Peter's visionary trance on the rooftop about eating unclean animals, which clashed with all his Jewish upbringing. Yet, aligning oneself with God's purposes can also involve a less direct and more evolving process which takes time and goes through several stages, as was the case, for example, with Nehemiah's vision to rebuild the walls of Jerusalem. That is, sometimes, and perhaps more often than not, God's message may not come – to use the expressive images from Elijah's story – in a "great and strong wind" or "earthquake" or "fire," but rather in "a still small voice" (1 Kgs 19:11–12; KJV),[3] and the material in the concluding chapters of this book is mostly concerned with how God's still small voice can be heard, interpreted, tested and implemented in contemporary Christian life. Having said that, we saw in Chapters 5 and 6 that even seemingly straightforward and direct divine messages need to be properly verified and appropriated, and therefore many of the following recommendations on how to discern, encompass and cultivate God's call will also be relevant to more "charismatic" visionary experiences.

---

3 Ensley (*Visions*, 45) puts it this way: "At times, the sacred invades us, lights flash, and bells ring. Most people experience dramatic visions from time to time. But this isn't the ordinary way. More frequently, we find ourselves moved by a special story someone tells us, or we are touched by a memory, a Scripture passage, a work of art, or a piece of music. Something is being said to us. What is it? It's the classic still, small voice by which God spoke to Elijah (1 Kgs 19:11–12 KJV)."

This emphasis on the less dramatic is consistent with the standpoint underlying the overall approach of this book, namely that the faculty of vision was opened up at Pentecost to *every* disciple, potentially enabling *every* Christian believer to tune into a Spirit-empowered visionary wavelength. Accordingly, while the Bible makes it clear that different people have different endowments – with some having unique prophetic gifting – the visionary capacity explored here will focus on the more *generic* ability of followers of Christ to utilise their inherent capacity to receive and behold divine vision to good effect.

What are the main features of an effective Christian vision?

We have seen in the previous chapters that a central feature of vision across the various applied domains is its *motivational potency*, that is, its capacity to act as a strong normative, directive or transformational force that can place individual people as well as whole communities or organisations on a new trajectory. The current discussion considers this motivational quality to be the main aspect of the "effectiveness" of a vision, with the three most important attributes of this motivational quality being *vivid clarity*, *arousing nature* and a balance between being *challenging but not unrealistic*:

- *Vivid clarity*. It was shown both in secular and biblical contexts (Chapters 2 and 4) that an effective vision needs to offer a clear, sensual picture of what success will look and feel like which is full of details and colours – the more elaborate a future image, the more likely it will become an effective motivating force. Accordingly, as we shall see in the next chapter, one of the best methods for strengthening Christian vision is to enhance the clarity and the vividness of the imagery involved.
- *Arousing nature*. A motivating vision needs to be of an emotionally stirring nature. Interestingly, when George Barna conducted interviews with visionary pastors in the US, there was a general agreement that a vision is "probably not from God if it does not excite you to the point that you occasionally find yourself being impatient with people, systems and situations."[4] The significance of the emotional quality of vision is also underlined in psychology (see Chapter 2), where it was demonstrated that imagining a scenario can evoke an emotional state that is as powerful as the experience of the same scenario in real life would be – the visionary, in effect, "pre-lives" the future experience and the feelings

---

4 Barna, *Power of Vision*, 92. As Stanley (*Visioneering*, 10) expressively puts it, with a motivating vision "The mundane begins to matter. The details, chores, and routines of life become a worthwhile means to a planned-for end." In a similar vein, Malphurs (*Developing a Vision*, 45) observes that when people start seeing what their churches could become, this vision elicits such strong emotions in them that at one point the "the vision is no longer a possibility but a must"; they discover that "they will never be satisfied until they are on the way to seeing the realization of their vision."

that are thus stirred up can act as a potent tonic. By way of illustration, Aubrey Malphurs recalls his own excitement at the birth of a vision as follows:

> In my personal experience I have felt a rush or flow of excitement. In that flash of time when it all comes together, there is a sense of having arrived. It feels right or clicks in such a way as to make the dreamer feel exhilarated. There is an extreme sense of ultimate accomplishment. The visionary walks away from the process knowing that he or she has reached a milestone in the ministry if not in his or her life.[5]

- *Challenging but not unrealistic.* Psychology has demonstrated that plausibility is an essential prerequisite for a motivating vision, since implausible images are likely to remain at the level of unregulated fantasy without any motivational response (see Chapter 2). This is, however, a possible point of contention when it comes to Christian vision: one may well argue that a God-ordained vision ought to take people *beyond* what they think they are capable of and also *beyond* the boundaries of their comfort zone, because a genuine Christian vision is not merely motivational but also *transformational*.[6] A verse of Scripture that has often been cited as an example of a biblical challenge for Christians to think big is Ephesians 3:20:[7] "Now to him who by the power at work within us is able to accomplish abundantly far more than all we can ask or imagine. . . ." The other side of the coin, however, is the concern that a vision should not be mixed up with fantasy; as David Hansen succinctly puts it, "if an image seems too good to be true, it probably is."[8] The ambiguity reflects the inherent tension between wishing to avoid unrealistic pipe-dreams or illusions on the one hand and not wanting to constrain God's purposes by channeling them into what appears realistic from a human perspective on the other; we shall come back to this

---

5 Malphurs, *Developing a Vision*, 91.
6 E.g. Barnett (*Reaching Your Dreams*, 6) suggests that the hallmark of a divine vision is that it is *oversized*: "The first test you can apply to your dream is: 'Is it too big for me to fulfil without God's help?' . . . If it's much bigger than you, you are on the right track." As Barnett then adds, "Your dream should be so big that it takes your breath away, makes you temporarily weak in the knees, and makes you cry out to God for help and guidance."
7 E.g. Malphurs and Penfold, *Re:Vision*, 157. Warren ("3 Aspects of Vision") paraphrases this verse as follows: "Think up the biggest thing you think I can do in your life, in your ministry, in your church – and I can top that. I can beat it."
8 E.g. Hansen, "Church of Your Dreams, 37. Barna (*Power of Vision*, 29) agrees: "Vision reflects a realistic perspective. Vision is not dreaming the impossible dream, but dreaming the most possible dream." Even Malphurs (*Developing a Vision*, 41) submits that an effective vision "drips with potential. It rests firmly on the bedrock of reality—thus it is highly feasible."

dilemma in the next chapter when discussing different ways of nurturing and strengthening one's vision.

What is vision like for the whole church community?

One important vision-related aspect in which churches differ from business organisations is that their core area of operation is far more uniform than the multiple enterprises on the marketplace; Shawn Lovejoy highlights this issue as follows:

> churches have a very unique challenge when it comes to vision. The visions for all churches come out of the same book! So it's impossible to have a completely "new" vision. The Bible even says it: "There is nothing new under the sun" (Eccl. 1:9).[9]

In a similar vein, Rick Warren submits that despite the variations in different church traditions, the core biblical mandate for every church involves fulfilling five fundamental purposes: worship, fellowship, discipleship, ministry and evangelism.[10] This raises the question of what the development of a "unique" vision should mean within an ecclesiastic context. Distinguishing two key dimensions of church life are helpful in this respect: the church's *culture* and *ministry*. The "culture" of an organisation refers to a set of emerging norms, values, beliefs and expectations that govern relationships and community life within the institution, and talking about church culture, Gilpin contrasts this aspect with the targets that make up the church's mission:

> My role as a visionary leader isn't primarily to declare where we'll all be in three years, but to declare what we'll all be like. God's word is much more to do with "culture creation" than with goal setting and actual, tangible accomplishments. God knows that creating a climate of the revelation knowledge of God is the context from which all growth will come.[11]

The kind of "culture creation" that Gilpin advocates represents a marked shift from looking only at the *outcome* of a vision to also envisaging the future *nature* and *character* of the church community.[12] Using the analogy

---

9 Lovejoy, *Vision*, 30.
10 Based on the Great Commandment, the Great Commission, Jesus' high priestly prayer (John 17) and Ephesians 4, and as illustrated in Acts 2; Warren, "How to Discern God's Vision."
11 Gilpin, *Confessions of a Confused Leader*, 24.
12 As Gilpin (ibid., 26) argues, "It's time to reinvent vision and see the eyes of your ministry and church refocused on 'culture', not just on outcome. God is up to something big – as we work according to our eyes of faith and with the language of hope, we'll surely see it all come to pass."

of a choir, this contrast can be likened to the conductor focusing mainly on the overall tone quality, balance and blend of the voices of the singers rather than on the pieces that the choir will eventually perform. Gilpin argues that visionary leaders need to be "cultural architects,"[13] and an important corollary of this perspective is to rely on specific people who embody the envisaged culture so that the whole church can embrace the dreams of these archetypical individuals for the overall collective vision.[14]

The other pole of the contrast, the outcome of the vision, can be viewed in concrete terms as specific *church ministries*, since these tend to be the primary vehicles for achieving goals in church contexts. We have seen earlier that vision is inextricably linked to "change," and therefore a new vision for a church will inevitably bring about a new ministry programme, often replacing existing ones that may have outlived their usefulness.[15] However, such a radical restructuring can realistically happen only if it is underpinned by a powerful new vision, and Hybels suggests that the essence of such a transformational vision be captured in "visionary pictures":

> For you it might be the picture of a hungry child being fed, her life being spared. It might be a picture of a homeless person finding shelter. It might be a picture of a dying church being revitalized or a lost person coming to faith or a volunteer finding a ministry that perfectly uses the gifts God has given. It might be a lonely person finding community or an artist finally using his creative gifts to serve God. There are as many life-giving, visionary pictures of the future as there are leaders among us.[16]

How can we generate a Christian vision?

Chapter 2 surveyed several psychological methods by which mental imagery can be consciously generated for various applied purposes, ranging from enhancing performance in sports and business to desensitising people with phobias. In these and other non-Christian applications, the powerful faculty of mental imagery is harnessed to good effect. Christian vision, however, differs from these approaches in a crucial aspect, namely that here the faculty of mental imagery is utilised for the purpose of connecting to *God's* communication channel in order to receive *divine* messages. This means

13 Gilpin, ibid., 140.
14 Sawyer ("Rekindling Vision," 62) offers a good illustration of how vision was rekindled in an established church by going along with the initiative of one of the members: "The truth is that for more than five years now, that church has had a successful preschool because it has had Jan Rea." As he concludes, "In rekindling vision, support people, not programs."
15 E.g. Schmidt ("Vision") argues, "The point of your church participating in the vision process is to help your church hear from God, identify those ministries that are no longer effective, and with the Lord's leading, determine new ministries to reach people."
16 Hybels, *Axiom*, 30.

that, strictly speaking, one cannot "generate" a divine vision but can only perceive it by God's grace – as Bill Johnson succinctly puts it, "revelation cannot be earned."[17] This was the understanding of divine vision even at the height of the movement of "cultivating" vision in the Middle Ages (see Chapter 5), since the various meditational techniques were not seen to guarantee visions but only to foster a sensitivity to their perception.[18] This being the case, the verb "generate" in the phrase "to generate vision" is rather a shorthand for three different processes: (a) to get into a receptive mindset/condition, (b) to discern God's call and (c) to appropriate/embrace the perceived vision. Let us examine these processes one by one.

Getting into a receptive mindset and creating appropriate conditions

Paul's visionary experience on the road to Damascus demonstrates that the desire to receive vision is not always a prerequisite for receiving it (since Paul's aspiration was not to hear from Jesus but rather to eliminate the followers of Jesus); yet, several verses of Scripture underscore the overall merits of actively seeking God's guidance: for example, Psalm 37:4 declares, "Take delight in the Lord, and he will give you the desires of your heart," and Proverbs 16:3 is even more explicit: "Commit your work to the Lord, and your plans will be established." The significance of a disposition of trust and reliance on God is also underlined by the assurance in Proverbs 3:5–6: "Trust in the LORD with all your heart and lean not on your own understanding; in all your ways acknowledge him, and he will make your paths straight." In the New Testament, people specifically asked Jesus, "What must we do to perform the works of God?" (John 6:28), and his answer was unequivocal: "This is the work of God, that you believe in him whom he has sent" (v. 29). That is, the primary condition for performing the plans that God has for believers is a mindset steeped in faith. Accordingly, Rahner maintains that the "abundance of grace enables us to call on God for help in our perplexity, to say to Him: Please give me what I am not able to accomplish! We can always do at least that much!"[19] In a similar vein, Malphurs maintains that the first step in aligning ourselves with God's purposes is to engage in "envisaging prayer," which should be an intentional, regular activity.[20] This was indeed the initial reaction of the biblical visionary Nehemiah: "When

---

17 Johnson, *Dreaming with God*, 133.
18 As Newman ("Medieval Visionary Culture," 3) explains, "Medieval teachers of meditation acknowledge the role of human striving, and encourage it, without assuming that assiduous spiritual effort will necessarily produce visions. But they do assert that such effort is often rewarded by divine grace. Judging from our extant sources, cultivated visions of this type were far more common than spontaneous ones."
19 Rahner, *Spiritual Exercises*, 284–285.
20 Malphurs, *Developing a Vision*, 72.

I heard these words I sat down and wept, and mourned for days, fasting and praying before the God of heaven" (Neh 1:4).[21]

Actively seeking God's call may not be effective if one does not create sufficient mental space for receiving the message; as Tommy Barnett argues, "One reason why people never discover their dream and purpose in life is because they never stop long enough to listen."[22] We saw in Chapter 1 that neuropsychology is unambiguous about the fact that we can experience mental imagery better in conditions which keep the distraction of external stimuli to a minimum, favouring an environment with limited background noise and luminance and where the imager is in a relaxed psychological state. This is in fact what Jesus himself selected for his communication with the Father: "In the morning, while it was still very *dark*, he got up and went out to a *deserted* place, and there he prayed" (Mark 1:35; emphasis added). Psalm 46:10 specifically calls for having quiet times with God – "Be still, and know that I am God!" – and Boyd echoes this call when he stresses that believers need regular quiet times when they "rest in an experience of Jesus as real."[23]

A passage in Isaiah offers further confirmation that getting into the right mental state is necessary for discerning and interpreting divine vision: Isaiah 28:7 declares that the priests and prophets who "reel with strong drink [and] are confused with wine . . . err in vision, they stumble in giving judgment." That is, staying sober and focused are necessary requirements for accurate discernment, and taking this together with the beneficial effects of a quiet, dark and relaxed environment, we may conclude that a certain amount of strategic acumen is instrumental to creating optimal conditions for receiving vision. Related to this is a report in 2 Kings 3:15 that when Elisha was requested to prophesy, he asked for a musician, and "while the musician was playing, the power of the Lord came on him." Newman notes in a similar vein that in order to foster visionary experiences, monastics developed several special meditational techniques that involved, for example, directing one's gaze towards a specific visual target (e.g. a crucifix),[24] often accompanied by fasting and ritual purification (as in Dan 10:3).[25] These suggestions,

21 Maxwell and Elmore (*Maxwell Leadership Bible*, 592) state about Nehemiah's prayer, "No doubt he got the vision and plan to rebuild the wall during his time of connection with God."
22 Barnett, *Reaching Your Dreams*, 9.
23 Boyd, *Seeing Is Believing*, 14. As Bill Johnson (*Dreaming with God*, 133) recommends, "Give God your nights," that is, dedicate the time when our mind is the quietest to God: "I try to end each day with my heart's affection stirred up and directed to the Holy Spirit. . . . The desire to give God our night season flows naturally from the child's heart that knows revelation cannot be earned. Ask Him specifically to minister to you in the night through visions and dreams."
24 Newman, "Medieval Visionary Culture," 15.
25 Hultgård, "Ecstasy and Vision," 220.

however, should be read together with the cautions about the potential dangers associated with cultivated vision, as discussed in Chapter 5.

Discerning God's call

How can we identify clues about the nature of God's specific call on us? This is a key question for the participants at Ignatian retreats (see Chapter 6), and it is noteworthy that even in the relatively controlled spiritual environment of such retreats there may be several markedly different pathways for receiving divine guidance, ranging from perceiving an explicit divine message to taking stock of one's options and performing rational cost-benefit calculations. This variety suggests that there may not be a single template to follow in such a quest, and therefore in order to discern God's call in full, one needs to consider a number of potential indicators. Indeed, Ensley reminds us that "Spiritual experiencing rarely comes in absolutely pure form, easy to discern and without any ambiguity. Our visions come in the midst of the struggles, desperations, yearnings, and imbalances of our lives."[26] This being the case, discerning God's purposes usually involves a sustained process of *vision-centred deliberation*, and this is true even when a person receives some form of a direct divine message: as seen in Chapter 5, even when God's revelation is seemingly unambiguous, the vision needs to be tested and properly interpreted. Following the broad principles set out by Ignatius for making an Election (see Chapter 6), we may identify four possible starting points for recognising cues about God's plan for us: a particularly meaningful *special event or experience*; a feeling of having a *burden* for something; conscious reflection on *available options and resources*; and a process that we may call "*visionary probing.*"

- *Special event/experience*. Sometimes, a specific incident, happening or encounter may give us initial guidance, or at least a "nudge," by triggering a response that is (perhaps unexpectedly) intense. Such events can be manifold, ranging from having a vision/dream or a prophetic message to more indirect means such as some verses of Scripture being "quickened up" when reading the Bible, thereby carrying a personal message;[27] witnessing a work of God (e.g. an exciting story of life transformation) as part of someone else's ministry, which ignites a strong reaction;[28] hearing a call for help that cuts right to the heart; or simply becoming aware of an untapped but highly promising opportunity[29] or a pressing problem that requires action (after all, as Stanley argues, "Every vision is a solution to a problem"[30]).

26 Ensley, *Visions*, 108.
27 Hybels, *Courageous Leadership*, 32.
28 Ibid., 33.
29 Malphurs, *Developing a Vision*, 66.
30 Stanley, *Making Vision Stick*, 25.

- *Feeling a burden.* Related partly to the previous point, a vision can begin with having a burden for a pressing issue, that is, a deep-seated concern that just would not let the person go. Experiencing strong frustration, sadness or even anger about a state of affairs is, according to Stanley, a candidate for a vision,[31] particularly if it reaches the intensity of a "moral imperative."[32] As he succinctly puts it, "Not all burdens are vision material. But every vision begins as a burden."[33] Hybels has coined the term "holy discontent"[34] to refer to the kind of profound dissatisfaction that feels more like divine frustration than subjective displeasure; such a disposition of a "deep dissatisfaction with what is and a deep, pressing desire for what they know could be"[35] is reminiscent of the biblical prophets' acute awareness of the "distress, pain, and dysfunction that are present in the community,"[36] which created a fertile ground for perceiving relevant vision.

- *Available options and resources.* One may start discerning God's call on one's life by rationally considering the full range of available options, weighing up the advantages, disadvantages and consequences associated with each. Such conscious deliberation may also include asking the question that Elisha put to a prophet's widow who came to him for help (2 Kgs 4:2): "Tell me, what do you have in the house?" Elisha then multiplied the little that the widow had (a jar of oil), and Barnett refers to this passage as an example of how one should consider one's talents, experiences and skills that have already been accumulated to build on when seeking God's vision.[37] To be sure, it is unlikely that such personal endowments should not be part of, in one way or another, God's overall plan for a person.[38] Such stock-taking may potentially lead to a "sense of destiny," that is, a feeling that this is the task that all who we are and what we have gone through so far has prepared us for.[39] In

---

31 Stanley, *Visioneering*, 17.

32 Ibid., 25.

33 Ibid., 20.

34 Hybels, *Axiom*, 19.

35 Malphurs, *Developing a Vision*, 67.

36 Brueggemann, *Theology of the Old Testament*, 625.

37 Barnett, *Reaching Your Dreams*, 172. As he argues, "Everybody has something, even if it's an idea, a strong body for labour, or a seemingly minor and mundane skill. Small things count when you are getting started on your dream. They can quickly become miracles and victories. Before Jesus fed the crowd, He asked how much food His disciples could round up. They found a pitifully small amount of fish and bread. . . . Within moments that small lunch fed thousands" (ibid.). Barnett even entitled an earlier book of his *There Is a Miracle in Your House*, and the subtitle of this work sums up his message: *God's Solution Starts with What You Have.*

38 E.g. Barna (*Power of Vision*, 150) submits, "Your personality, your past experiences and your context for ministry will converge to result in a ministry that is uniquely you and that is important in the overall growth of God's work on Earth."

39 Stanley, *Visioneering*, 42.

fact, Gilpin extends this point to the whole church context, arguing that "The key to your church's growth lies not in the realm of the miraculous, but within the dust of the people who already surround you."[40] This is consistent with Paul's teaching in Romans 12:4–8 that believers are endowed with unique giftings, talents and abilities, all of which are necessary for the overall operation of the body of Christ – hence the need for a collective vision.

- "*Visionary probing.*" The conscious deliberation described earlier needs to be tested to see whether the desired outcome reflects more than merely a human incentive or endeavour (see later for further discussion on testing one's vision), and this validation process may be augmented by the power of mental imagery through envisaging some of the short-listed options in the mind's eye. If one of these envisaged options feels more natural or evokes deeper feelings in us, or alternatively, if one of the images sticks with us and we find ourselves daydreaming about it later, this might be a clue that we are on the right track. Lonsdale gives the example of Ignatius himself to illustrate this point: before Ignatius launched his ministry, envisaging himself as a romantic hero caused pleasant immediate emotions in him but ultimately left him "feeling sad and dissatisfied."[41] On the other hand, the mental pictures of serving God – even ones that included difficulty and pain – led him to experience "deep feelings of joy which left him satisfied and cheerful."[42]

Having described the previous options as four separate starting points can easily give the (wrong) impression that they represent alternative routes that exclude each other. In many cases this is not true: during the sustained process of aligning oneself with God's plans, all the four options might well come into play, acting as confirmation or further clarification for each other.[43] Indeed, Rahner makes an important point in this respect when he explains that "the intervention of heaven has often given either the first idea or the last impulse for the execution of something which in other ways and for weightier reasons was already recognized as correct, useful and necessary."[44]

---

40 Gilpin, *Confessions of a Confused Leader*, 44.
41 Lonsdale, *Eyes to See*, 93.
42 Ibid.
43 The following practical suggestion by Munroe (*Principles and Power of Vision*, 60) reflects the interconnected nature of these points: "Take half an hour and allow yourself to dream about what you would like to do in life. What ideas and desires do you have? What have you always wanted to do? Think about your primary gifts or talents. How do your dreams and your gifts go together? Write down your ideas, desires, and gifts and read them over every evening for a week. Then ask yourself, 'Do these ideas hold true? Are they what I want to do?' "
44 Rahner, *Visions and Prophecies*, 29.

Appropriating and embracing God's call

In order to transform the initial stimulus/burden/inspired decision into a mature vision, we need to *appropriate* and *embrace* God's call. This requires above all ongoing *prayer* to unlock the details of the divine plan – as Maxwell and Elmore summarise, prayer "infuses the vision, enabling us to see what God wants to do."[45] We already saw the significance of "envisaging prayer" as part of getting into a receptive mindset, and we shall see later that an ongoing, intensive prayer life is also indispensable throughout the duration of bringing the vision to fruition for ensuring that we remain on God's path and for sustaining the visionary momentum. At the appropriation stage, an extended period of prayer is needed because it "internalizes the burden, deepening our ownership of a need."[46] It is significant to note in this respect that after the Apostle Paul received his vision, he did not discuss it with any human being for as long as three years:

> But when God, who . . . called me through his grace, was pleased to reveal his Son to me . . . I did not confer with any human being, nor did I go up to Jerusalem to those who were already apostles before me, but I went away at once into Arabia, and afterwards I returned to Damascus. Then after three years I did go up to Jerusalem to visit Cephas. . . .
>
> (Gal 1:15–18)

The use of some rare Greek vocabulary for what is translated as "confer" and "human being" in this passage instead of some more obvious and seemingly appropriate words is particularly interesting in this respect (although this point is lost in the NRSV translation): Paul appears to deliberately emphasise the fact that he did not rely on external human interpretation of his vision but spent an extensive period by himself working out the divine meaning and implications.[47]

Prayer not only matures the vision but also creates a visionary context to fine-tune the initial perception. The first discernment usually contains only the main theme of the vision, and Warren explains that after this "what"

---

45 Maxwell and Elmore, *Maxwell Leadership Bible*, 592.
46 Ibid.
47 The Greek word for confer (*prosanatithēmi*) appears only twice in the New Testament, and Dunn ("The Relationship Between Paul and Jerusalem," 462) points out that its meaning in NT Greek "does not simply mean 'consult with someone' in general, but has the more technical sense of consulting with someone who is recognized as a qualified interpreter about the significance of some sign – a dream, or omen, or portent, or whatever." This unique meaning is complemented with the phrase to which Paul links this word, "*sarx kai haima*," which literally means "flesh and blood" and which only occurs in the Bible four other times, typically used, according to Douglas Moo (*Galatians*, 105), "to set up a contrast with something divine."

component one needs to wait to find out the "how" and the "when" elements.[48] Without sufficiently appropriating God's calling, we also run the danger of meeting opposition too early, at a stage when one is still ill-prepared to properly protect the vision.[49] Therefore, as will be elaborated in a separate section later, we need to resist any impatient desire to move from decision to action prematurely. Indeed, Psalm 37:7 declares, "Be still before the LORD, and wait patiently for him," and the prophet Habakkuk could not have been any clearer about this point:

> For there is still a vision for the appointed time;
>   it speaks of the end, and does not lie.
> If it seems to tarry, wait for it;
>   it will surely come, it will not delay.
>
> (Hab 2:3)

Taking ownership of someone else's vision

In the discussion of collective vision at the end of Chapter 6, it was mentioned that it is not always the church leader who is the author of a vision, because visions may originate from a variety of sources – the leader's main responsibility is to take ownership and become the *chief carrier* of the vision. The need to take ownership of someone else's vision is even more important for people who are not in a leadership position but who "buy into" the collective vision of a church or a ministry. In some cases people may find their own personal dreams within the larger vision and thus become vision partners proper. In some other cases, however, one needs to serve what is, in effect, someone else's dream. Barnett argues that not only is this possible, but that in fact it is an inevitable step in reaching one's own vision: "It's an iron law of leadership that you don't attain authority until you have served someone else's dream."[50] As with any good service, he explains, the secret of doing it well is to be selfless and to give it one's best shot, as if it was one's own vision, considering it a learning experience with lessons that will help to fulfil one's own dream.[51]

48 Warren, "3 Aspects of Vision."
49 E.g. Stanley (*Visioneering*, 75) warns, "when God first lays something on your heart for you to do, don't tell anybody. To begin with, nobody is going to be nearly as excited as you are. Their lack of zeal has the potential to shut you down before you get started. To share a vision prematurely usually guarantees a less than warm reception."
50 Barnett *Reaching Your Dreams*, 119; as he adds, "I can point to literally dozens of ministries that were started at my church by people who first served my dream. After a while, God gave each a unique dream and the opportunity to carry it out. Today at least half a dozen such ministries have gained national prominence and are touching thousands, even hundreds of thousands, of lives."
51 Ibid., 120.

How can we be sure that the vision is from God?

While the previous guidelines for identifying clues about a divinely inspired vision can provide initial orientation, they cannot guarantee that the outcome of the deliberation process will be fully aligned with God's purposes.[52] We saw in Chapter 5 that there is no watertight procedure to verify an authentic vision and therefore we have to accept that similar to how "we know only in part, and we prophesy only in part" (1 Cor 13:9), we also perceive and behold vision in part. Stanley is right that not every good idea is a God idea,[53] and it is important for this reason in particular to embed the vision in a context of ongoing prayer. We have seen in previous chapters that the need to submit one's plans and desires to God in prayer is a recurring message in the Scriptures, and that this has been at the heart of the different approaches to receiving God's vision throughout the centuries, from the mystics of the Middle Ages to contemporary Ignatian spirituality. Thus, Lonsdale's conclusion about Ignatius's teaching has broader relevance:

> Decision-making on a particular occasion by discernment of spirits pre-supposes a living relationship with God and a background of daily life in which I am trying to be responsive and faithful to the Spirit's leading. That is the only context in which Ignatius' guidelines have meaning and use. And a "right" decision about a course of action I should take is . . . what appears to be the best in the circumstances and is the expression of the deepest truths of ourselves within the setting of this day-to-day relationship with God.[54]

In addition to a dynamic prayer life in general, we may also receive more specific reassurances that we are on the right track by means of a number of *validity checks* of our visionary idea along the lines of the authentication principles described in Chapter 5 and the procedures of Ignatian discernment in Chapter 6:

- *Tests of content and consequence.* Some inappropriate ideas and options can be discounted straight away through checking the content of a

---

52 E.g. Aschenbrenner (*Stretched for Greater Glory*, 190) highlights in this respect that even Ignatius himself was deceived by two spontaneous inner experiences that initially appeared to be holy. As described in Ignatius's *Autobiography*, during an early period of his life when his daily routine was centred around prayer and penance, Ignatius's sleep was regularly disrupted by "great illuminations and spiritual consolation," making him "lose much of the time he had set aside for sleep." Later in his life, when he was supposed to do more studying, his learning of Latin grammar was disrupted by experiencing strong "new light on spiritual things and new delights." As Aschenbrenner sums up, Ignatius realised in both cases through prayerful reflection that they were actually temptations meant to deflect him from his God-ordained course of action.

53 Stanley, *Visioneering*, 25.

54 Lonsdale, *Eyes to See*, 109.

visionary message to see if it is in harmony with biblical truths. Then, in the spirit of telling the tree by its fruit (Matt 12:33), an examination of the hoped-for consequences of the vision-inspired idea constitutes a second effective layer of filter. Here the key questions to ask are whether the vision will bring glory to God (rather than to someone else) and whether the desired outcomes will contribute to the advancement of the kingdom of God (rather than to some other cause).

- *Test of strength*. The initial tests of content and consequence are helpful for screening out ideas that are not entirely biblical, but they will be less effective when it comes to deciding whether an idea that *could* potentially be from God is really so.[55] One indication of the God-inspired nature of a vision is the powerful hold that it can have on the receiver, so that he/she simply cannot let it go. Barnett puts it this way: "A God-given dream is a bothersome thing: it won't leave you alone! It keeps bobbing to the surface of your heart, clamouring for your mind's attention. If that's how your dream behaves, then it is probably from God."[56]
- *Test of emotions*. Another way of separating from the many fleeting ideas and desires going through our minds the one that originated with God, or which he approves of, is to examine our own deep feelings carefully. In his *Spiritual Exercises*, Ignatius linked the discernment as to whether an experience is from the good spirit or the evil spirit to gauging what fills our hearts: sadness and anxiety or peace, joy and love.[57] According to John Futrell, "Ignatius' constant use of the words contentment, satisfaction, peace, tranquility, quiet, and rest to describe the experience of confirmation refer to the psychological dynamism that bears interior testimony that one has judged rightly."[58] The subjective experience of deep-seated joy is often a principal sign of being closely aligned with God's purposes.[59]
- *Test of time*. The saying "time will tell . . ." carries particular relevance for the authentication of a vision. As Williamson contends, "if a true vocation has been received to serve God . . . a testing time of waiting is often to be expected . . . [offering] an indication of whether the call has

---

55 Stanley (*Visioneering*, 25) puts the dilemma as follows: "We all have good ideas. Everybody is concerned or burdened about something. But how do you know which ideas to act on?"

56 Barnett, *Reaching Your Dreams*, 6. Malphurs and Penfold (*Re:Vision*, 155) add, "If it's God's vision, you will be passionate about it. If you feel strongly and care deeply about the vision, then likely it is God's vision and captures your heart."

57 E.g. *Spiritual Exercises*, 315.

58 Futrell, "Ignatian Discernment," 63.

59 In Barna's (*Power of Vision*, 92) interview survey of American pastors who have experienced vision, a recurring observation was that they sometimes reached "a state of euphoria about the prospects that may result from the vision." As he adds, "This, in itself, was a new experience for some of these men because they were not particularly emotional beings. Yet, the force of the vision was something that caused them to overflow with feeling about the potential and the impact of having the vision become a reality."

been genuine and whether commitment to it is unwavering."[60] If an idea is indeed from God it will not fade away, and this knowledge can be useful for reducing people's anxiety that they might miss their call.

- *Test of collective response.* Many if not most Christian visions also require the active involvement of others besides the visionary. It was argued in Chapter 6 that developing a collectively shaped vision is an essential aspect of such team projects, and this aspect of vision can also be utilised for the purpose of external verification as described in Chapter 5. Sharing the vision with a select group of trusted people and then asking them to appraise its authenticity might not only provide invaluable validity feedback but it can also lead to receiving intercessory prayer support. Moreover, because – as argued before – "People support what they help to create," the team may eventually evolve into the core of a larger grouping of collective visionary partners (see Chapter 8).

How long do we need to wait before starting to implement a vision?

The question of how long one needs to wait before setting the vision in motion is an important one, because the obvious answer – namely, that one should begin as soon as God's call has been sensed – is usually *incorrect*. Contemporary writers on vision repeatedly stress the point that a freshly perceived vision rarely requires immediate action, and in fact, a premature start may not only be ineffective but can even cause damage[61] – for example, Malphurs and Penfold submit that "Premature action can be as debilitating as failure to act at all."[62] What is needed is patience, which is not easy when someone feels that he/she has heard from God. Nevertheless, the significance of patience is repeatedly highlighted in the Scriptures: it is mentioned as part of the fruit of the Spirit (Gal 5:22) and also in lists of Christian virtues (e.g. 2 Cor 6:6; Col 3:12); it is a corollary of love (1 Cor 13:4); and Hebrews 6:12 declares that faith and patience are prerequisites for inheriting God's promises. The need to wait for the Lord is also one of the recurring themes in the Psalms (e.g. Ps 27:14; 37:7, 9, 34; 62:1; 130:5–6), and Lamentations 3:25 affirms that "The Lord is good to those who wait for him, to the soul that seeks him."

---

60 Williamson, *Ezra, Nehemiah*, 175. Stanley (*Visioneering*, 20) argues similarly: "Time allows us to distinguish between good ideas and visions worth throwing the weight of our life behind. . . . After all, if what concerned you yesterday is of little concern today odds are that was not vision material."

61 E.g. Stanley (*Visioneering*, 20), states: "I have witnessed a good many people with what seemed to be God-ordained visions charge out of the starting gates too early. And the result is always the same. Failure. Discouragement. Disillusionment. A vision rarely requires immediate action. It always requires patience."

62 Malphurs and Penfold, *Re:Vision*, 38.

Patience is thus frequently contrasted in the Scriptures with the human urge to follow one's own timing and impulse, and the importance of a period of waiting is also evident in the lives of some of the prominent biblical visionaries. Regarding Paul, we have already seen that after his revelation of Jesus Christ on the road to Damascus he spent several years preparing before launching his ministry (Gal 1:15–18), and Nehemiah also devoted several months to private intercession before the opportunity arose to present his request to the Persian king. With respect to Moses, although the Old Testament says little about his early passion to deliver the slave-nation of Israel to freedom, Malphurs and Penfold rightly point out that according to Acts 7:25, he had this vision long before his escape from Egypt (with Heb 11:24–27 corroborating this), and after his initial, ill-conceived attempt to do something about it (i.e. killing an Egyptian; Acts 7:26–28; Exod 2:11) he spent 40 years as a resident alien in the land of Midian before God's timing came.[63] Recall also that Abraham waited for 25 years for the child of promise to be born, Joseph spent years in prison and David was on the run from King Saul in the wilderness for almost a decade, and we may agree with Barnett that "Every hero in the Bible went through lengthy times of delay."[64]

What explains the necessary waiting period prior to the implementation of a vision? Proverbs 19:2 states that "Desire without knowledge is not good, and one who moves too hurriedly misses the way," suggesting that the risk of premature engagement lies in acting without sufficient knowledge and information. This supports Rick Warren's observation (discussed earlier) that divine revelation appears gradually, starting with the main theme and followed later by details of the how and when.[65] Indeed, the Bible contains some dramatic examples of untimely implementation going very wrong: Michael Duncan reminds us in this respect of Abraham's attempt to accomplish God's vision with human ingenuity by sleeping with a handmaid and fathering Ishmael (Gen 16) and of King David's efforts to bring the Ark of the Covenant back to Jerusalem by his own method (2 Sam 6:1–10), and Peter's desire to keep Jesus from Calvary (Matt 16:22–23) may also be seen as an example of how human schemes can go against God's plan.[66] Proverbs 19:21 addresses this issue head on: "Many are the plans in a person's heart, but it is the Lord's purpose that prevails" (NIV).

Stanley suggests that besides the need to fully appropriate the details of God's plan, waiting can also serve two additional purposes. First, the maturation period may be needed for the vision to "survive in the real world."[67] We have seen that the essence of vision is change, and change is often perceived by people as inherently challenging; thus, the vision needs

---

63 See Malphurs and Penfold, *Re:Vision*, 37.
64 Barnett, *Reaching Your Dreams*, 208.
65 Warren, "3 Aspects of Vision."
66 Duncan, *From Vision to Victory*, 25–26.
67 Stanley, *Visioneering*, 21.

to be well-developed "before being exposed to the cynical, critical, stubborn environment in which it is expected to survive."[68] We may also add here that the waiting period does not only allow the vision to mature but it may also be instrumental to maturing the visionary him/herself. Second, during the time of preparation, God will be working in the background, preparing the way by adjusting the circumstances, raising necessary helpers and creating opportunities.[69] In Nehemiah's case, for example, a divine opening was needed for Nehemiah to be able to present his request to the king, and after several months of praying, his opportunity arrived suddenly when the king asked about the reason for his sadness (Neh 2:2). Kouzes and Posner offer several case studies of thriving vision-inspired contemporary Christian ministries whose birth was reminiscent to that of Nehemiah's project in that it involved lengthy periods of waiting and preparation.[70] In the next chapter we shall consider several concrete strategies that can be employed during the incubation period to prepare for the realisation of the vision.

So, when is the right time to start implementing a vision? In Barna's survey of vision-led ministries in the US, the time period taken to gain clarity on the initial vision varied considerably, often lasting many months.[71] There simply does not appear to be a hard and fast rule about when the untimely becomes opportune and appropriate, which foregrounds the principle in Ignatian spirituality that the Election is incomplete until it has been submitted and confirmed by God (see Chapter 6). According to this principle, the right time to start implementing a vision is when one receives a metaphorical "divine green light" in some way. The accurate discernment of being released to act, however, might well turn out to be the most difficult aspect of receiving God's call, particularly because there is some undeniable tension between two conflicting positions in this respect: on the one hand, the considerations outlined earlier favour patience over the human urge to do it now; on the other hand, there is a compelling argument in favour of stepping out in faith even when not everything is completely clear-cut. Maxwell, for example, reasons that when someone receives a vision, the resources are never fully available to accomplish it and, yet, at that point "God expects us to begin walking in obedience according to the dream He has given us."[72] He believes that God does not move before we move first, and cites the miraculous feeding of the multitudes as an illustration of this point, when

68 Ibid. Warren ("Rick Warren's Challenge") argues in a similar way: "Vision is a very fragile thing. . . . It shrinks when it gets wet from criticism."
69 Stanley, *Visioneering*, 24.
70 For example, in the case of the Society of St. Andrew – a Christian hunger-relief organisation in the US that has salvaged since 1983 500 million pounds of food that would have been wasted otherwise – Kouzes and Posner ("Five Practices of Exemplary Leadership," 8–11) report that it took the founders three years of fairly constant prayer for their initial idea to be translated into action.
71 Barna, *Power of Vision*, 87.
72 Maxwell and McManus, "Turning Vision Into Reality."

Jesus told the disciples who turned to him for solving the seemingly insoluble problem, "You give them something to eat" (Mark 6:37). Maxwell thus concludes, "Your resources to fulfil the dream will come during the last step of the dream,"[73] and Gilpin, following Jonathan's example in 1 Samuel 14:6,[74] also advocates this stance: "Why don't we just give it a go? It's a noble task and it's possible that we just might succeed!"[75] As Gilpin argues, the goal is to "create a 'yes' culture, where it's a 'yes' until God says no: it's a green light unless we see a red light."[76] Indeed, many would agree with Warren's caution that undue patience might carry a real danger:

> You may be overflowing with vision for your ministry, but there is a point where you have to stop thinking about it and talking about it, and instead, start doing something about it – moving your vision toward a tangible reality. I've met thousands of pastors with incredible vision for ministry in their community, but sadly they never got past the thinking stage.[77]

Summary

The notion of "vision" embraced in the current chapter has integrated three different understandings: mental imagery as discussed in psychological theories, divine communication as used in the Bible and a motivational future scenario as introduced in sport psychology and business management. It was argued that such a broadly conceived Christian vision has numerous practical implications, and the material in this chapter was centred around generating such a vision in Christian believers by suggesting ways of discerning God's call and then aligning themselves with it. It was argued that while a divine call is sometimes direct and striking, in many other cases receiving a vision fully involves a subtle and gradual process of perceiving, interpreting, testing and implementing it. From an individual's perspective,

---

73 Ibid. Maxwell also adds, "God gives us resources according to our dreams and according to our obedience. . . . God has never given anybody a dream that He did not want that person to fulfil. He has never given a dream that could be fulfilled at step one. So start walking, be obedient, and watch God fulfil that dream in your life."

74 1 Sam 14:6: "Jonathan said to the young man who carried his armour, 'Come, let us go over to the garrison of these uncircumcised; it may be that the Lord will act for us; for nothing can hinder the Lord from saving by many or by few.'"

75 Gilpin, *Confessions of a Confused Leader*, 16.

76 Ibid., 26.

77 Warren, "How to Start." Elsewhere Warren ("3 Aspects of Vision") adds, "I have what I call Polaroid vision. Have you ever taken a Polaroid picture? You take it and the longer you look at it the clearer it gets. That's true in my life. When I first started Saddleback, I didn't know what it was going to end up like. All I knew was that God had called me to this spot and I had a bunch of ideas in a bag and I wanted to build it on the five purposes of God. As I have walked with the Lord and worked with the Lord over the years, the vision has gotten clearer and clearer."

an effective Christian vision involves a vivid and arousing image of an attractive, God-ordained future state, which requires taking a challenging but not impossible route to reach it; vision for a whole church is more specifically concerned with two key aspects of the church's future life, its culture and its ministries.

Of course, a divine revelation cannot be consciously "earned," and therefore the phrase "generating vision" is rather a shorthand for three different processes: to get into a receptive mindset, to discern God's call and to appropriate and embrace the perceived vision. The receptive mindset includes both a desire to hear from God and sufficient mental space for receiving that call, which can be created by regularly spending quality time in God's presence in an environment that excludes visual distractions and loud noises. As for discerning God's call, we may identify four possible starting points for recognising cues about God's plan for us: a particularly meaningful special event or experience; the feeling of having a burden for something; conscious reflection on available options and resources; and "visionary probing," that is, envisaging some of the shortlisted options in our mind's eye. Then, in order to transform the initial stimulus, burden or inspired decision into a fully-fledged vision, we need to embrace and appropriate God's call. This requires ongoing prayer, which helps to fine-tune the initial perception and which also matures the visionary him/herself.

Not every good idea coincides with God's specific plan for a person, and humans can perceive and behold vision only in part; this again foregrounds an intensive and dynamic prayer life to ensure that one does not go off at a tangent. In addition, we can receive specific reassurances that we are on the right track by means of a number of validity checks on various aspects of the perceived vision and our reaction to it: tests of content, consequence, strength, emotions, time and collective confirmation from others. However, even if our vision-inspired idea "passes" these tests, this does not automatically mean that we need to act upon it immediately; a premature and hasty start may not only be ineffective but can even cause damage. Instead, we need to wait patiently for the Lord to equip us with the necessary details, maturity and means, and to prepare the ground by adjusting the circumstances, rousing necessary helpers and creating opportunities. One of the most difficult aspects of discerning a divine vision is to sense when one is ready to step out and start acting on it; this is made more difficult by the tension between, on the one hand, not wanting to rush into things, and, on the other, not wanting to miss God's call by acting too timidly.

References

Aschenbrenner, George A. 2004. *Stretched for Greater Glory: What to Expect from the Spiritual Exercises*. Chicago: Loyola Press.
Barna, George. 2009. *The Power of Vision: Discover and Apply God's Plan for Your Life and Ministry*. Ventura, CA: Regal.

Barnett, Tommy. 1993. *There's a Miracle in Your House: God's Solution Starts with What You Have*. Lake Mary, FL: Charisma House.

Barnett, Tommy. 2005. *Reaching Your Dreams: 7 Steps for Turning Dreams into Reality*. Lake Mary, FL: Charisma House.

Boyd, Gregory A. 2004. *Seeing Is Believing: Experience Jesus through Imaginative Prayer*. Grand Rapids, MI: Baker Books.

Brueggemann, Walter. 1997. *Theology of the Old Testament: Testimony, Dispute, Advocacy*. Minneapolis, MN: Fortress.

Duncan, Michael. 2014. *From Vision to Victory: The Nehemiah Project*. Marston Gate: CreateSpace.

Dunn, James D. G. 1982. "The Relationship between Paul and Jerusalem According to Galatians 1 and 2." *New Testament Studies* 28: 461–78.

Ensley, Eddie. 2000. *Visions: The Soul's Path to the Sacred*. Chicago: Loyola Press.

Futrell, John Carroll. 1970. "Ignatian Discernment." *Studies in the Spirituality of Jesuits* 2, no. 2: 47–88.

Gilpin, Dave. 2006. *Jesus, Save Me from Your Followers: Confessions of a Confused Leader*. Chichester: New Wine Press.

Hansen, David. 1997. "Church of Your Dreams." In *Renewing Your Church through Vision and Planning: 30 Strategies to Transform Your Ministry*, edited by Marshall Shelley, 35–41. Minneapolis, MN: Bethany House.

Hultgård, Anders. 1982. "Ecstasy and Vision." *Scripta Instituti Donneriani Aboeniensis* 11: 187–200.

Hybels, Bill. 2002. *Courageous Leadership*. Grand Rapids, MI: Zondervan.

Hybels, Bill. 2008. *Axiom: Powerful Leadership Proverbs*. Grand Rapids, MI: Zondervan.

Johnson, Bill. 2006. *Dreaming with God: Co-Laboring with God for Cultural Transformation*. Shippensburg, PA: Destiny Image.

Kouzes, James M., and Barry Z. Posner. 2004. "The Five Practices of Exemplary Leadership." In *Christian Reflections on the Leadership Challenge*, edited by James M. Kouzes and Barry Z. Posner, 7–38. San Francisco: Jossey-Bass.

Lonsdale, David. 2000. *Eyes to See, Ears to Hear: An Introduction to Ignatian Spirituality*. London: Darton, Longman and Todd.

Lovejoy, Shawn. 2016. *Be Mean About the Vision: Preserving and Protecting What Matters*. Nashville, TN: Thomas Nelson.

Malphurs, Aubrey. 2015. *Developing a Vision for Ministry*. 3rd ed. Grand Rapids, MI: Baker Books.

Malphurs, Aubrey, and Gordon E. Penfold. 2014. *Re:Vision: The Key to Transforming Your Church*. Grand Rapids, MI: Baker Books.

Maxwell, John C., and Tim Elmore. 2007. *The Maxwell Leadership Bible*. Nashville, TN: Thomas Nelson.

Moo, Douglas J. 2013. *Galatians*. Grand Rapids, MI: Baker Academic.

Munroe, Myles. 2003. *The Principles and Power of Vision: Keys to Achieving Personal and Corporate Destiny*. New Kensington, PA: Whitaker House.

Newman, Barbara. 2005. "What Did It Mean to Say "I Saw"? The Clash between Theory and Practice in Medieval Visionary Culture." *Speculum* 80, no. 1: 1–43.

Rahner, Karl. 1963. *Visions and Prophecies*. Translated by Charles H. Henkey and Richard Strachan. Freiburg: Herder.

Rahner, Karl. 1967. *Spiritual Exercises*. Translated by Kenneth Baker. London: Sheed and Ward.

Sawyer, Dennis. 1997. "Rekindling Vision in an Established Church." In *Renewing Your Church through Vision and Planning: 30 Strategies to Transform Your Ministry*, edited by Marshall Shelley, 59–67. Minneapolis, MN: Bethany House.

Schmidt, J. David. 2000. "So You've Got a Vision – Now What?". *Enrichment Journal (on-line)* 5, no. 1.

Stanley, Andy. 1999. *Visioneering: God's Blueprint for Developing and Maintaining Vision*. Colorado Springs, CO: Multnomah Books.

Stanley, Andy. 2007. *Making Vision Stick*. Grand Rapids, MI: Zondervan.

Warren, Rick. 2016. "How to Discern God's Vision for Your Church." In *Pastors. com*. https://pastors.com/discern-gods-vision-church/.

Warren, Rick. 2017. "3 Aspects of the Vision God Has for Your Church." In *Pastors.com*. https://pastors.com/3-parts-of-vision/.

Warren, Rick. 2018. "How to Start Growing toward Your Vision This Year." In *Pastors. com*. https://pastors.com/how-to-start-growing-toward-your-vision-this-year/.

Warren, Rick. 2011. "Rick Warren's Challenge to the SBC Pastors' Conference." In *Pastors.com*. https://pastors.com/rick-warrens-challenge-to-the-sbc-pastors-conference/.

Williamson, H. G. M. 1985. *Ezra, Nehemiah*. Word Biblical Commentary 16. Dallas, TX: Word Books.

8 Vision in the Christian life II
Cultivating the perceived vision

The previous chapter outlined several possible avenues for generating a Christian vision, arguing that when the yearning to discern God's calling is accompanied by a prayerful and patient disposition, believers can receive divine vision through their innate imagery faculty that was activated by the release of the indwelling Spirit at Pentecost. However, the discussion also highlighted a deep-seated tension between wishing to avoid unrealistic pipe-dreams and not wanting to constrain God's purposes by channeling them into what appears realistic from a human perspective. The current chapter takes this dilemma as its starting point and begins with an examination of the inherent limitations of human efforts to behold divine vision. We shall see that the process of realising such visions is usually riddled with challenges and setbacks, but at the same time, if handled wisely, obstacles can be overcome by perseverance and mistakes can have a maturing effect. Psychological research offers a number of lessons in this respect concerning ways of nurturing and strengthening mental imagery, and the following discussion will present several practical strategies to cultivate vision in a principled manner. Let us begin the discussion by considering a general observation of leadership experts and visionary leaders, namely that "vision leaks."

Vision leaks

Contemporary church leaders and leadership experts converge in their belief that, in John Piper's words, "The vision that God put in [us], that got everybody fired up, leaks out."[1] For example, an often mentioned estimate is that it may take as little as one month for a congregation to forget a vision if it is not reiterated again and again,[2] and within the Bible the process of an initial holy zeal fading away is specifically mentioned about the church in Ephesus: as Lovejoy notes, this church was started and nurtured by the

---

1 Cited in Duncan, "Casting Vision"; see also Hybels, *Courageous Leadership*, 44; *Axiom*, 52; Lovejoy, *Vision*, 49; Malphurs, *Developing a Vision*, 38; Maxwell, *Laws of Leadership*, 159; Stanley, "Vision Leaks"; Warren, "Rick Warren's Challenge."
2 E.g. Malphurs, *Developing a Vision*, 107.

Apostle Paul himself, yet within a generation it is mentioned in Revelation as a community which has abandoned its first love (Rev 2:6).[3] The waning of the passion evoked by a vision can be partly explained by the corroding effects of the everyday demands of busy lives, in a similar way to how the "cares of the world and the lure of wealth choke the word" (Matt 13:22) in Jesus' Parable of the Sower.[4] Part of the reason, however, is also related to certain constraints inherent to the nature of human motivation in general: it is well known in psychology that motivation is never constant but shows continuous ebbs and flows, and unless it is regularly refueled, it loses momentum and peters out with time.[5] The motivational quality of divine vision is particularly subject to such a decrease, because a vision-inspired project often feels like an uphill enterprise that goes against all odds – as Stanley has found, "From the outset, just about every God-ordained vision appears to be impossible."[6]

The seeming impossibility of a vision-inspired project is related to the fact that the participants are likely to be under-equipped for at least some aspects of the visionary task,[7] and that the vision usually requires them to be stretched beyond not only their comfort zones but also beyond what they think are the limits of their capabilities – all in all, success appears to be out of reach and beyond their strength.[8] As a result, there will be times when they experience deep fatigue and discouragement in the same way as even prominent visionaries are described in the Bible; for example, we read in Numbers 11:11–15 that at one point Moses got so exhausted and, quite frankly, fed up with his task of leading the stiff-necked Israelites that he cried out to God:

> Why have you treated your servant so badly? Why have I not found favour in your sight, that you lay the burden of all this people on me? Did I conceive all this people? Did I give birth to them, that you should say to me, "Carry them in your bosom, as a nurse carries a sucking child," to the land that you promised on oath to their ancestors? . . . I am not able to carry all this people alone, for they are too heavy for me. If

---

3 Lovejoy, *Vision*, 59.
4 As Hybels (*Axiom*, 52) expressively summarises, "Something 1 have to remind myself of constantly is that people in our churches have real lives. . . . They have challenging jobs, children to raise, lawns to mow, and bills to pay. Because of all these daily responsibilities, the vision we poured into them on Sunday begins to drain out of them sooner than we think."
5 See, e.g. Dörnyei and Ushioda, *Teaching and Researching Motivation*, 60; Dörnyei et al., *Motivational Currents*, 80.
6 Stanley, *Visioneering*, 41.
7 E.g. Stanley (ibid., 154) sums up a familiar situation as follows: "If you are honest . . . it is true: You don't have the necessary experience. You don't have the financial resources to see your vision through to completion. You don't have the necessary skills. You have no formal education in this particular field. People have tried this before with no success."
8 E.g. Stanley (ibid., 42) aptly concludes, "The task always appears to be out of reach. And the reason it appears that way is because it is. God-ordained visions are always too big for us to handle. We shouldn't be surprised. Consider the source."

this is the way you are going to treat me, put me to death at once – if I have found favour in your sight – and do not let me see my misery.

Similarly, in Nehemiah's project of building up the walls of Jerusalem, there came a point when Nehemiah was confronted with defeatist attitudes: "The strength of the burden bearers is failing, and there is too much rubbish so that we are *unable* to work on the wall" (Neh 4:10; emphasis added). Paul also hit some very low points during his ministry (see e.g. 2 Cor 7:5–6; Phil 1:23; 2 Tim 4:16), and his summary of the catalogue of hardships he had to endure beggars belief:

> Five times I have received from the Jews the forty lashes minus one. Three times I was beaten with rods. Once I received a stoning. Three times I was shipwrecked; for a night and a day I was adrift at sea; on frequent journeys, in danger from rivers, danger from bandits, danger from my own people, danger from Gentiles, danger in the city, danger in the wilderness, danger at sea, danger from false brothers and sisters; in toil and hardship, through many a sleepless night, hungry and thirsty, often without food, cold and naked. And, besides other things, I am under daily pressure because of my anxiety for all the churches.
>
> (2 Cor 11:24–28)

The fact that even biblical heroes can go weary resonates with Stanley's observation that "Many visions die in the time between what and how. . . . When *how* seems out of sight, it is tempting to put *what* out of mind."[9] Indeed, he concludes, "At some point it is just easier to lower your sights, jettison your vision, and shoot for a target you have some hopes of hitting."[10] Yet, Moses, Nehemiah and Paul all managed somehow to persevere and run the race to the end, achieving the vision that God lay on their hearts. Where did they find the strength to do so and, more generally, how can the leakage of vision be stopped and the "vision bucket" refilled? There is no single answer to these questions, but rather there are several possible ways to cultivate a vision through gaining strength, building confidence, enhancing the imagery, dealing with obstacles, promoting perseverance and self-control, learning from setbacks, envisaging and fine-tuning a roadmap, and finally, soliciting support from vision partners.

Gaining strength

The Bible is laced with verses of encouragement and exhortation related to strength. People are repeatedly urged to be strong[11] and are reassured that it

---

9 Ibid., 56.
10 Ibid.
11 E.g. Deut 31:6; 2 Sam 10:12; Ps 31:24; Isa 35:3–4; Zech 8:9, 13; 1 Cor 16:13; Eph 6:10; 2 Tim 2:1; Jas 5:8.

is the Lord who gives strength to his people[12] – in fact, it is mentioned more than once that human strength in itself is futile.[13] Taken together, these passages point believers to turning to God in prayer at times of exhaustion and lethargy, a message that is expressively articulated in Isaiah 40:29–31:

> He gives strength to the weary
>   and increases the power of the weak.
> Even youths grow tired and weary,
>   and young men stumble and fall;
> but those who hope in the LORD
>   will renew their strength.
> They will soar on wings like eagles;
>   they will run and not grow weary,
> they will walk and not be faint. (NIV)

Psalm 105:4 (repeated in 1 Chr 16:11–12) encapsulates the essence of Isaiah's message as "Seek the Lord and his strength; seek his presence continually," and the promise of divine strengthening is pronounced several times in the Scriptures.[14] Accordingly, Munroe suggests that prayer is the primary tool which "sustains us in the demands of vision. . . . Prayer is the essential resource of vision,"[15] and indeed, Paul offers a prayer to this effect in Colossians 1:9–11: "For this reason, since the day we heard it, we have not ceased praying for you and asking that you may be . . . made strong with all the strength that comes from his glorious power [literally, power of glory], and may you be prepared to endure everything with patience. . . ." A few verses later in the same letter Paul further explains that it is God's strength that drives him – "For this I toil and struggle with all the energy that he powerfully inspires within me" (1:29) – and in Philippians 4:12–13 his message is even more explicit: "In any and all circumstances I have learned the secret of being well-fed and of going hungry, of having plenty and of being in need. I can do all things through him who strengthens me." Lastly, in 2 Timothy 4:17–18, Paul directly links the divine fortification to the objective of accomplishing the vision he has received (i.e. to proclaim the good news to the Gentiles):

> But the Lord stood by me and gave me strength, *so that* through me
> the message might be fully proclaimed and all the Gentiles might hear

---

12 E.g. Ps 18:32; 68:35; 89:21; 1 Chr 29:12; Isa 58:11; Ezek 34:16; Hab 3:19; Luk 24:49; Acts 1:8; Col 1:9; Phil 4:13; 2 Tim 4:17; 1 Pet 4:11; 5:10.
13 E.g. Deut 8:17–18; 1 Sam 2:9; Ps 33:16; 147:10.
14 E.g. Isa 58:11: "The Lord will guide you continually, and satisfy your needs in parched places, and make your bones strong; and you shall be like a watered garden, like a spring of water, whose waters never fail." See also Ps 18:31–32; 29:11; 68:35.
15 Munroe, *Principles and Power of Vision*, 213.

it. So I was rescued from the lion's mouth. The Lord will rescue me from every evil attack and save me for his heavenly kingdom. (emphasis added)

Regarding Nehemiah, when his building project in Jerusalem came to a particularly low point, he, too, turned to the Lord for strength: ". . . for they all wanted to frighten us, thinking, 'Their hands will drop from the work, and it will not be done.' But now, O God, strengthen my hands" (6:9). God answered his prayer and the walls of Jerusalem were completed in as little time as 52 days; as Nehemiah recounted, "when all our enemies heard of it, all the nations around us were afraid and fell greatly in their own esteem; for they perceived that this work had been accomplished with the help of our God" (6:16). This was thus a perfect example of the principle stated in 1 Peter 4:11: "whoever serves must do so with the strength that God supplies, so that God may be glorified."

Finally, we are told about Moses that he considered himself inadequate to fulfil God's calling to perform the task of rescuing the Israelites from Egyptian slavery (Exod 3:11; 4:1, 10, 13), and his outburst to God (cited earlier) also indicates that he never stopped feeling stretched beyond his limits, even after Pharaoh finally allowed the Israelites to leave. How did he manage to keep going? He talked to God honestly and God responded, "I will be with you" (3:12), a promise he later reiterated, "My presence will go with you, and I will give you rest" (33:14). The history of the journey to the Promised Land evidences that gaining sufficient strength to continue after each setback was far from easy, but God kept reassuring Moses, "Is the Lord's power limited? Now you shall see whether my word will come true for you or not" (Num 11:23). Moses stuck to his belief that he declared at the beginning of his first song, namely that "The Lord is my strength and my might" (Exod 15:2), and in his final speech to the Israelites he reaffirmed this trust: "Be strong and bold; have no fear or dread of them, because it is the Lord your God who goes with you; he will not fail you or forsake you" (Deut 31:6).

Bolstering confidence – "the battle belongs to the Lord . . ."

The story of Moses shows that even someone who received direct and regular communication from God could struggle with insufficient confidence in his ability to realise the vision he was entrusted with. To be sure, practically speaking the odds were stacked against him, as they were against David when he faced Goliath or against King Jehoshaphat when he faced a mighty army invading his country. As is well known, David fearlessly confronted Goliath, declaring that "the battle is the Lord's and he will give you into our hand" (1 Sam 17:47). In contrast, King Jehoshaphat was initially scared, but he chose to trust the Lord and turned to him for help: "Jehoshaphat was afraid; he set himself to seek the Lord, and proclaimed a fast throughout all Judah. Judah assembled to seek help from the Lord" (2 Chr 20:3). God heard the Israelites' plea and reassured them through an oracle by the prophet Jahaziel, which again emphasised that the battle was his: "Do not fear or be dismayed at this great multitude; for the battle is not yours but God's" (v. 15). As a result, Jehoshaphat declared to his people, "Believe in the LORD your God and you will be established; believe his prophets" (v. 20), and subsequently a great victory followed. Significantly, in both crisis situations the main source of human confidence was the knowledge that *the battle belongs to the Lord*, and Proverbs 21:31 reiterates this message: "The horse is made ready for the day of battle, but the victory belongs to the Lord."

It is important to note that attributing the outcome of the battle to the Lord does not shift all responsibility to God, because the proverb cited above stipulates that the horse needs to be "made ready." Similarly, God's pronouncement to King Jehoshaphat also contained the instruction that the Israelites should take up their position: "Tomorrow go down against them . . . take your position, stand still, and see the victory of the Lord on your behalf" (2 Chr 20: 16–17). In other words, winning the battle requires human preparation, initiation and taking up an adequate fighting position; the conclusion of God's message to Jehoshaphat and his army reiterates the injunction to step out: "Do not fear or be dismayed; tomorrow go out against them, and the Lord will be with you" (v. 17). Raymond Dillard points out that this message is consistent with the template provided in Deuteronomy for a speech to be delivered by a priest before battle:[16]

> Before you engage in battle, the priest shall come forward and speak to the troops, and shall say to them: "Hear, O Israel! Today you are drawing near to do battle against your enemies. Do not lose heart, or be afraid, or panic, or be in dread of them; for it is the Lord your God who goes with you, to fight for you against your enemies, to give you victory."
>
> (20:2–4)

Moses also applied this "winning formula" at the Red Sea before Pharaoh's troops caught up with his people: "Do not be afraid, stand firm, and see the deliverance that the Lord will accomplish for you today. . . . The Lord will fight for you, and you have only to keep still" (Exod 14:13–14).

Thus, the message that people should not lose heart because the battle is for God to fight appears in the Bible as many as five times, repeatedly underlining the fact that when God's people are acting in accordance with his will, they should gain confidence from remembering this promise. In desperate situations it may be admittedly difficult to do so, and in Moses's case, for

16 Dillard, *2 Chronicles*, 158.

example, we are told that even after this reassurance people kept manifesting insufficient faith by pleading for help, which solicited a rather brusque response from God: "Why do you cry out to me? Tell the Israelites to go forward" (v. 15) – that is, "Stop whining and get on with it." We should realise, however, that this message was more than a mere rebuke as it presented a highly effective strategy to combat fear; as Barnett explains, "Fear is a sinister, dream-depriving force. Fear keeps some people from taking the first steps toward their dreams. . . . Here's how I conquer fear: instead of spending a lot of time anticipating the battle, I get to the battle quickly. I would rather be in the fight than waiting for it to start!"[17]

Enhancing the vision

Psychological research has accumulated a wealth of knowledge on how mental imagery can be intensified, and several established strategies can also be applied to the cultivation of divine vision. Of course, the enhancement of Christian vision cannot involve the bolstering of the stimulus at its source, because this source is the sovereign Lord, but the process of beholding the vision may be reinforced at the recipient's end. The fact that our human capacity in this respect may be wanting was already pointed out by Augustine of Hippo in his *Confessions* when he concluded the description of a mystical experience he had had in Milan as follows:

> But I did not possess the strength to keep my vision fixed. My weakness reasserted itself, and I returned to my customary condition. I carried with me only a loving memory and a desire for that of which I had the aroma but which I had not yet the capacity to eat.[18]

The following four vision-enhancement strategies may be used to good effect with regard to Christian vision: *sharpening the imagery; reactivating the vision regularly; not losing sight of the alternative;* and *celebrating success.*

- *Sharpening the imagery* is based on the recognition that a mental image (regardless of its source) may not be effective as a motivator of action if it does not have a sufficient degree of elaborateness and vividness; as discussed in the previous chapter, images with insufficient specificity and detail will fail to evoke a significant motivational response. So, how can we add vivid colours and tangible details to a desired future scenario? Psychology suggests that an effective way of elaborating on vision is to mentally visit and revisit the envisaged scene regularly, thereby gaining

17 Barnett, *Reaching Your Dreams*, 60. Warren ("How to Start") makes the same point: "The first step is always the hardest. What should you do when you know something is God's will but you're scared to do it? You do it anyway!"
18 Augustine, *Confessions*, VII. xvii (23) (pp. 127–128).

further familiarity with it and thus expanding the depth of one's imagined experience. Most imagery-training programmes start by getting the
participant to visualise in the mind's eye a familiar location – often one's
bedroom – and then, over several weeks, the trainee is encouraged to
gradually add further details to the scene and to start manipulating it,
for example by moving the furniture around. Actively immersing in an
envisaged scene is not unlike gospel meditation (discussed in Chapter 6),
with the difference being that here the destination of our virtual wander-
ing is not a biblical scene (as in gospel meditation) but the God-inspired
future vision. This approach can therefore be likened to imaginative
prayer (Chapter 6) that is directed at an imaginary target. Maxwell is
right that "Imagination is the soil that brings a dream to life,"[19] and
Munroe builds on this principle when he recommends the following
practice:

> God gave us the gift of imagination to keep us from focusing only
> on our present conditions. He wants us to take a "tour" of our
> visions on a regular basis. What do you imagine doing? Go on
> a tour of your dream. Visit everything. Check it out. See all the
> details. Notice its value. Then come back to the present and say,
> "Let's go there. God!"[20]

• *Reactivating the vision regularly* has already been mentioned in the section on vision leakage, referring to how people tend to forget a vision
  they have heard (and possibly even subscribed to) relatively quickly
  unless it is recast repeatedly.[21] The essence of this strategy is to regularly
  reboot the vision in order to save it from being overrun by the myriad
  of other competing interests and life concerns.[22] In other words, in order
  to ensure a successful outcome, the vision needs not only to be generated but also to be consciously *kept alive* through regular reminders.
  These may include taking frequent "virtual tours" in the mind's eye (as

19 Maxwell, *Put Your Dream to the Test*, xix.
20 Munroe, *Principles and Power of Vision*, 93.
21 E.g. according to Malphurs and Penfold (*Re:Vision*, 161), "Most vision casters agree that it
    takes only about a month for people to forget the vision. The general rule is to repeat it over
    and over every day in a different way. This will be a primary responsibility of the pastor."
22 The need for such a reactivation practice is explained by the nature of the self-concept. Self-
    knowledge is such a complex entity that it cannot be active in one's mind as a whole at any
    time but only in part, and the continually shifting array of available active self-knowledge,
    "the self-concept of the moment" (Markus and Wurf, "Dynamic Self-Concept," 306),
    has been termed the "working self-concept." Because the various self-images, including
    the desired future ones, have to compete for recognition in the limited mental space of
    the working self-concept, they need to be reactivated at regular intervals (see e.g. Henry,
    "Dynamics of Possible Selves," 89–90).

discussed earlier) or having regular vision-related events and celebrations that prime and evoke the vision as a kind of "déjà vu of the future."[23]

• *Not losing sight of the alternative.* It was argued in Chapter 2 that vision exerts maximum motivational impact if people also have a vivid image of what the *alternative* would be, that is, a picture of the potential negative consequences of failing to achieve the desired end-state. The pushing power of these feared images will effectively complement the pulling power of the desired target. Therefore, "rocking the boat" (Chapter 2) – that is, not only making the "there" attractive (by the vision) but also the "here" intolerable (through describing the alternative) – may be necessary to create sufficient *dissonance* to warrant a change. We saw in Chapter 4 that the practice of using the complementary functions of contrasting positive and negative imagery was a common biblical practice exercised by the prophets to engender transformation, and Rahner points out that even in an Ignatian retreat (Chapter 6), the first week is designed in such a way that it should make the participants "mistrustful" of their former life so that this would then stir them to make a decision.[24] Finally, Stanley urges us never to forget the fact that although God does have a vision for our lives, it is not inevitable that this will be fully realised; as he expressively concludes, "Missing out on God's plan for our lives must be the greatest tragedy this side of eternity."[25]

• *Celebrating success.* Celebration can be defined as a joyous event to applaud something positive, and the usual understanding of celebrating success is that it takes place at the completion of a project. It can, however, also be held *during* the course of implementation of a vision in order to report *progress* towards accomplishing the vision's targets. In such cases, the celebration may not only boost morale but can also be an effective means to further clarify the vision and to intensify its implementation.[26] According to Lovejoy, this is partly due to the implicit message that such a celebration communicates (given that people tend to celebrate things that they value and attach importance to) and partly because it demonstrates that "we're winning."[27] People like to be on the winning side, not only because of the experience of sharing the victory but also because success is seen as a sign that their work is not in vain. Moreover, the successful unfolding of a project can also be interpreted as the hallmark for God's involvement; Nehemiah successfully silenced

23 Dörnyei and Kubanyiova, *Motivating Learners*, 108.
24 Rahner, *Spiritual Exercises*, 126.
25 Stanley, *Visioneering*, 14.
26 E.g. As Hybels (*Axiom*, 52) explains, "when you wrap a little real-life proof around the accomplishment of your church's vision and show that the dream really is coming true, the fog will start to clear and people's heads will start to nod. 'Oh yeah!' they'll suddenly remember. 'I get it! I get it! This is what we're about! This is why we exist as a church.'" See also Stanley, *Making Vision Stick*, 39.
27 Lovejoy, *Vision*, 76.

his first critics by simply stating, "The God of heaven is the one who will give us success" (2:20), and the celebration of success affirms this point.

Dealing with obstacles and failure

A critical aspect of cultivating a Christian vision is to find the right way of dealing with external obstacles and attacks, and to process setbacks and failure constructively. If the various difficulties that a vision-inspired initiative encounters are not handled well, those can not only undermine and even halt the entire project, but can also bring overwhelming discouragement to the people involved, often driving them from the particular ministry or church. The almost inevitable experience of setbacks is due to a combination of the demanding nature of the tasks involved in a Christian vision, the unavoidable gaps in the initial action plan, the typically insufficient resources, the participants' limited time and energy to commit to the project as well as their lack of the necessary experience and skills for at least some aspects of the job. The vision is also likely to encounter direct opposition, both human and spiritual. Human opposition stems partly from the fact that vision involves change and thus an alteration of what people are used to, and partly from individual differences in how people expect things to proceed in an area they care deeply about. Spiritual opposition occurs because by contributing to the advance of the kingdom of heaven, Christian ministries unavoidably incur into "enemy territory," thereby activating forces to try to disrupt the work of God. Indeed, when Jesus sent out his disciples on their first missionary outreach (Matt 10), he made it clear that their mission would take them on a collision course with hostile forces of various sorts.[28] So, let us address some common contemporary issues in this respect, along with methods of dealing with them in order to sustain the visionary momentum.

Criticism and hostile opposition

Criticism is the first and probably most common challenge facing any vision. It is common because, as Stanley summarises, visions are "easy to criticise" – in fact, visions "attract criticism" and are "difficult to defend against criticism" – and as a result, visions "often die at the hands of the critics."[29] When Nehemiah started the building work in Jerusalem, the project elicited a great deal of reproach and condemnation from influential adversaries, and the taunting, heavily sarcastic questions his opponents asked concerned every aspect of the work: "What are these feeble Jews doing? Will they restore things? Will they sacrifice? Will they finish it in a day? Will they revive the stones

---

28 See e.g. Dörnyei, *Progressive Creation*, 255–258.
29 Stanley, *Visioneering*, 141.

out of the heaps of rubbish – and burned ones at that?" (Neh 4:1–2). The final mockery summed it all up: "That stone wall they are building – any fox going up on it would break it down!" (v. 3). Thus, Nehemiah's adversaries implied that the builders were frail (with a unique Hebrew word used in the text that literally means "withering" or "without hope"[30]), the building materials were substandard and the final outcome was poorly constructed and pitifully weak. Significantly, therefore, the criticisms shrewdly attacked the most vulnerable aspect of any vision by suggesting that it was no more than an unrealistic human fantasy or pipe-dream.[31] How did Nehemiah respond? Not by defending himself or by arguing the points raised, and neither did he confront his opponents with his royal authority; rather, he turned to prayer and asked God to take care of those who wanted to obstruct the divine purpose (Neh 4:4–5).[32] By not dealing with the criticism himself but leaving it to God, he also avoided a common detrimental shift that Stanley warns about, namely the drift from being vision-centred to critic-centred.[33]

The Apostle Paul was also subject to constant criticism and mockery; as Raymond Brown summarises,[34] he was dishonoured, given a bad reputation and treated as an impostor (2 Cor 6:8); he was "opposed and reviled" (Acts 18:6); his bodily presence was ridiculed and his speech was deemed "contemptible" (10:10); and in Athens he was called a "babbler" and was "scoffed" at (Acts 17:18, 32). He, too, resisted taking action himself, and simply moved on: as described in Acts, he "left them" (17:33) and "in protest he shook the dust from his clothes" (18:6). This was consistent with the advice given by Jesus to his disciples: "If anyone will not welcome you or listen to your words, shake off the dust from your feet as you leave that house or town" (Matt 10:14) and "When they persecute you in one town, flee to the next" (v. 23). Hostile criticism, however, was not everything that Paul had to endure. The Book of Acts and in his epistles (e.g. 2 Cor 6:4–5; 11:23–33) describe a catalogue of additional afflictions, including arrests, imprisonments, physical beatings, lashings, being stoned and left for dead. He was also shipwrecked several times and suffered from illnesses. Yet, we have seen earlier that Paul managed to find renewed strength in God, and in his letter to the Galatians he urged the readers to persevere: "So let us not grow weary in doing what is right, for we will reap at harvest time, if we

---

30 See e.g. Levering, *Ezra and Nehemiah*, 141.
31 Williamson (*Ezra, Nehemiah*, 216) points out that the second and third questions are worded in a somewhat obscure manner, but together they "ridicule the suggestion that God can be cajoled into prospering the work as if by the wave of a magic wand." The final two questions are consistent with this tone as they imply that "that the Jews are hopelessly overoptimistic: the task is larger than they suppose, and it will take longer than they have calculated."
32 Myers, *Nehemiah*, 141;
    Williamson, *Ezra, Nehemiah*, 106.
33 Stanley, *Visioneering*, 151.
34 Brown, *Message of Nehemiah*, 59.

do not give up" (6:9). Let us explore further the foundations of this "holy perseverance."

Self-control and role modelling

The endurance required for fulfilling one's calling has been expressively captured in several places in the Scriptures by the metaphor of an athlete running the race to the end;[35] for example in his second letter to Timothy, Paul concludes about his life, "I have fought the good fight, I have finished the race, I have kept the faith" (4:7). According to 1 Corinthians 9:25–27, the key factor in being able to finish the race is *self-control*:

> Athletes exercise self-control in all things; they do it to receive a perishable wreath, but we an imperishable one. So I do not run aimlessly, nor do I box as though beating the air; but I punish my body and enslave it, so that after proclaiming to others I myself should not be disqualified.

Self-control is an important human attribute that is generally seen in psychology as a key aspect of any purposeful, strategic behaviour.[36] It was a well-known concept in New Testament times, as it was considered a principal virtue by Greek philosophers such as Socrates, Plato, Aristotle and the Stoics.[37] The notion appears in the Bible in several senses within the broad semantic domain of self-discipline/self-regulation/self-mastery,[38] and it is presented as an essential human quality for the followers of Christ; for example, in Galatians 5:23 it is listed as part of the fruit of the Spirit[39] and in 2 Timothy 1:7 it is listed alongside power and love: "for God did not give us a spirit of cowardice, but rather a spirit of power and of love and of self-discipline." The significance of self-controlled restraint was also mentioned in the Old Testament wisdom literature as a vital aspect of being victorious (e.g. Prov 16:32), and it is emphasised that the absence of self-control can ruin a person: "They [the wicked] die for lack of discipline, and because of their great folly they are lost" (5:23; see also 25:28).

The key characteristic of the biblical portrayal of self-control from our current perspective is that it is presented as an attribute that believers should consciously strive for (1 Thess 4:3–5; 1 Pet 1:13; 4:7; 2 Peter 1:4–5). This

---

35 E.g. 1 Cor 9:23–27; Acts 20:24; 2 Tim 4:7; see also Gal 5:7; Phil 3:14; Heb 12:1.
36 Contemporary psychology sees self-regulation as one of the key determinants of human behaviour; see e.g. Vohs and Baumeister, *Handbook of Self-Regulation*.
37 E.g. Betz, *Galatians*, 288; Gordon, "Self-Control," 386; Longenecker, *Galatians*, 263.
38 E.g. self-control (*enkrateia* and cognates like *enkrateuomai* and *enkratēs*), self-discipline (*sōphronismos* and cognates like *sōphrosynē* and *sōphroneō*), steadfastness (*hypomonē*) as well as lack of self-control or incontinence (*akrasia*) and being temperate (*nēphalios*).
39 Betz (*Galatians*, 288) rightly points out that its position at the very end of the list of the various facets of the Spirit's fruit is a marked one, as it stands in juxtaposition to love, the first item in the list.

implies that it is *trainable*, because if being disciplined could not be cultivated, believers would not be urged to make every effort to acquire it. The passage by Paul cited earlier confirms this by likening the mastery of self-control to how athletes prepare for competitions, and in Titus 2:2–6, Titus is encouraged to *teach* both men and women of various age groups to be self-controlled. Yet, despite these exhortations, the Scriptures offer no explicit instruction on how this can be achieved, as illustrated, for example, in Paul's farewell to the Ephesian Elders before leaving for Jerusalem:

> I served the Lord with great humility and with tears and in the midst of severe testing by the plots of my Jewish opponents. . . . However, I consider my life worth nothing to me; my only aim is to finish the race and complete the task the Lord Jesus has given me – the task of testifying to the good news of God's grace.
>
> (Acts 20:19–24; NIV)

Paul clearly considered promoting perseverance to be critical for his legacy to the church, nevertheless he does not offer any specific strategies to follow. Instead, what he does offer is *himself as an example* to imitate. This is a powerful approach, referred to in psychology as *role modelling*, and it is known for being able to exert considerable influence in shaping individuals' values, attitudes and beliefs.[40] Paul was fully aware of the significance of setting a personal example and he repeatedly mentions this in his epistles. In 2 Thessalonians 3:7–9 he writes (regarding supporting oneself through work), "For you yourselves know how you ought to follow our example. . . . We did this . . . in order to offer ourselves *as a model for you to imitate*" (emphasis added). In Philippians 3:17, he is even more explicit about the general relevance of role modelling: "Brothers and sisters, join in imitating me, and observe those who live according to the example you have in us." Then, in 1 Corinthians 1:16–17 he reiterates this theme:

> I appeal to you, then, be imitators of me. For this reason I sent you Timothy, who is my beloved and faithful child in the Lord, to remind you of my ways in Christ Jesus, as I teach them everywhere in every church.

Finally, in 2 Corinthians 6:4 he specifically "commends" himself "in every way," and Guthrie points out that this act of "commending himself" is a "vitally important thread that has been woven through the book (3:1; 4:2;

---

40 In his classic book on social learning theory, Canadian psychologist Albert Bandura (*Social Learning Theory*, 12) submits that "virtually all learning phenomena resulting from direct experience occur on a vicarious basis by observing other people's behaviour and its consequences for them." People continually and actively search for models they perceive as representative of what they wish to achieve, and doing so, Bandura concludes, "guides and motivates self-development" (p. 88).

5:12; 7:11; 10:12, 18; 12:11), one that lies at the heart of the apostle's intentions for 2 Corinthians."[41] What Paul does, in effect, is present himself as "an apostolic ideal,"[42] and highly significantly for the current discussion, the very first attribute he mentions in this context, is "*great endurance*, in afflictions, hardships, calamities, beatings, imprisonments, riots, labours, sleepless nights, hunger . . ." (vv. 4–5; emphasis added). Paul's perseverance did indeed have a profound impact on his contemporaries, and his reputation lived on after him, as evidenced by a letter written by the apostolic father Clement at the end of the first century in which he underscored the virtue of endurance in his description of Paul.[43]

Consistent with the biblical mandate, the significance of perseverance and role modelling in pursuing a vision has also been emphasised with regard to contemporary Christian leadership. Barna, for example, concludes that "The most important factor is to pursue His vision doggedly. Do not let the wear and tear of the process defeat you,"[44] and Malphurs and Penfold's argument about the impact of such a commitment on Christian ministries echoes the points made earlier concerning Paul: "The leader's life communicates the ministry's vision. He must live the vision. He must personify the dream. This happens when he models the vision."[45] Indeed, Kouzes and Posner do not hesitate to state that "The most powerful thing a leader can do to mobilize others is to set the example . . . by walking the talk."[46] Using different words, Hybels contends the same principle: "Wise leaders understand that the single greatest determinant of whether followers will ever own a vision deeply is the extent to which those followers believe the leader will own it."[47]

Processing failure

Barnett recounts a personal story that is likely to resonate with many readers because it occurs in many forms and variations:

> When we were looking to buy a building for the church in Los Angeles, I felt as if everything were against me. I was certain it was God's will for

41 Guthrie, *2 Corinthians*, 325.
42 Harris, *Second Corinthians*, 470.
43 See Best, *Second Corinthians*, 60–61.
44 Barna, *Power of Vision*, 88.
45 Malphurs and Penfold, *Re:Vision*, 161.
46 Kouzes and Posner, "Five Practices of Exemplary Leadership," 12; they then reiterate, "Leading by example is how leaders make visions and values tangible." In a similar vein, McAllister-Wilson ("Shared Vision," 65) submits that "Leaders teach vision constantly, sometimes with words and sometimes through rich nonverbal and symbolic forms of communication" and Maxwell (*Put Your Dream to the Test*, 128) succinctly states, "People buy into the dreamer before they buy into the dream."
47 Hybels, *Axiom*, 35; he then adds, "Your followers take their cues from you. They will only sacrifice for the vision if you will. They will only take a bullet for the cause if they believe down to their toes that you would do the same" (ibid).

us to buy a certain old waterworks building and turn it into our facility. But a company came and bought it out from under us at the last minute. I was devastated. Then we found a bigger building for about the same price, and I became convinced it was for us. But the city council said they didn't want us to use the building for a church. I was greatly disappointed, to say the least. In the end, we found a much bigger building that allows us to do vastly more ministry. It is better in every way. But before we found that building, I had to fight through the disappointment of losing the first two.[48]

In similar stories, the initial failed building purchases may be replaced with business bankruptcies, unsuccessful church plants, doomed career choices or any other botched attempts to accomplish something that one thought would be right in the sight of God. Stories like this beg the question: if God wanted people to have the final positive outcome, why did they have to go through a series of initial failures rather than being led directly to what was destined for them? There can be many possible answers; in Barnett's case, for example, there may have been something wrong with the first two buildings; or the third building was not available at the beginning and God was working on releasing it; or Barnett and his team needed the experience of the first two failures to fully appreciate the third option; or the first attempts were ahead of God's timetable for some other reason, etc. Barnett himself interpreted such false starts as follows: "God uses failures to educate us. Mistakes and success are partners; they work together."[49]

It is impossible to second-guess what may lie behind a particular failed attempt, but one may gain comfort from Paul's declaration in Romans that "*all* things work together for good for those who love God, who are called according to his purpose" (8:28; emphasis added). The problem often is, however, that our human interpretation of what the "for good" element involves does not coincide with God's intention; after all, Romans also contains a verse that states that "suffering produces endurance" (5:3), and yet few people would willingly choose to suffer because they believe that it is "good" for them. Nevertheless, James 1:3–4 not only reiterates this principle but also tells believers to consider trials "nothing but joy":

> My brothers and sisters, whenever you face trials of any kind, consider it nothing but joy, because you know that the testing of your faith produces endurance; and let endurance have its full effect, so that you may be mature and complete, lacking in nothing.

It would appear, therefore, that at least sometimes one can *grow* during a period in the wilderness, and indeed, according to Psalm 119:71, failure

48 Barnett *Reaching Your Dreams*, 56.
49 Ibid., 45.

experiences may be beneficial: "It is good for me that I was humbled, so that I might learn your statutes." This may explain Stanley's observation that there are times when every visionary must swallow his/her pride and revise his/her plan,[50] and in fact, Stanley submits that he has never met or heard of anyone "who accomplished anything significant for the kingdom who didn't have to revise plans multiple times before the vision became a reality."[51] This observation is consistent with the calamities that many biblical visionaries suffered (discussed earlier). In Nehemiah's case, for example, at one point the builders not only got tired and discouraged but also came under a death threat from their adversaries. Yet, Nehemiah did not abandon the vision but dealt with the trouble: he reorganised the work by setting up a system of guarding the workforce, which slowed down progress in the short term but allowed for the walls to be completed in the end.

Envisaging a roadmap

The survey of psychological theories explaining the motivational impact of vision in Chapter 2 highlighted the significance of a detailed action plan to accompany vision, because it is the concrete pathway of tasks and strategies leading to the desired future state that distinguishes a motivationally relevant vision from empty daydreams or fantasies. Indeed, Warren speaks from decades of experience when he advises church leaders: "Remember that nothing becomes *dynamic* until it becomes specific. When a vision is vague, it holds no attraction. The more specific your church's vision is, the more it will grab attention and attract commitment."[52] Maxwell argues in a similar vein that the problem with some "big visions" such as "taking my city for Christ" is that they are not linked to any specific strategies to pursue. As such, they may create excitement for a week or a month but will then peter out: "we must have a strategy and a process to make our vision become a reality. Many pastors fail to see God's vision fulfilled because they never have a strategy for fulfilling that vision."[53]

The point made by Maxwell is crucial: sometimes a vision fails to be realised not because of a lack of wanting but rather because of lacking the understanding of the process needed to reach the envisaged target. Even when someone has a clear idea about a desired end-state and is fully set to reach this outcome, the vision only becomes productive if it is accompanied by a concrete

---

50 Stanley, *Visioneering*, 159.
51 Ibid., 158.
52 Warren, "6 Ways to prevent Vision Drift"; he then the adds, "Part of reminding your congregation about the church's vision is to continually put before them the activities that will help the church achieve the vision. If part of your vision is to help people build meaningful relationships in your church, remind your people of the vision as you encourage them to get involved in small groups. If part of your vision is to be involved in local and global missions, regularly communicate opportunities for them to participate in missions."
53 Maxwell and McManus, "Turning Vision Into Reality."

roadmap, that is, a blueprint which maps out action pathways that will lead to it. Research in educational psychology corroborates this experience: for example, Daphna Oyserman and her colleagues have concluded in a study – whose title says it all: "Seeing the Destination but Not the Path" – that it was not the lack of aspiration that contributed to the low school attainment of the participating students from disadvantaged socioeconomic backgrounds, because many participants *did* possess internal images of their successful future selves; instead, the major factor contributing to their low school attainment was an unclear understanding of how to achieve their aspirations.[54]

Thus, an indispensable aspect of cultivating people's initial vision is to help them to "see the path" leading to it. The following two strategies can facilitate this process both for individual believers and for whole church communities and ministries:

- Using "*process imagery*." It has been found in psychology that sometimes even when people have good intentions, they may fail to achieve their goals. One lesson drawn from such cases has been that it promotes successful goal completion more when people are encouraged to focus on the *journey* to the goal rather than merely on the final outcome itself.[55] The concept of *process imagery* builds on this strategy by adding sensory details to the action plan; that is, it involves mentally mimicking the experience of progressing towards the final vision.[56] For example, in an influential study, Shelley Taylor and her colleagues showed that students who envisioned the steps leading to a successful goal achievement performed considerably better than those who focused exclusively on the targets they wanted to reach.[57] In other words, the vivid details that are necessary for bringing a vision alive (Chapter 7) should not be limited only to the image of the projected future but should also include aspects of the roadmap leading up to it. This implies the need for prayerful meditation on available options and possible directions to follow (for individuals), and painting a vivid picture of the journey towards the vision in the vision statement (for church leaders).
- *Breaking down the project into bite-size tasks for everybody.* A fundamental principle of goal-setting theory is that for greater effectiveness, long-term goals need to be broken down into a series of shorter-term targets or "subgoals."[58] Having a list of such manageable "action-

54 Oyserman, Johnson and James, "Seeing the Destination but Not the Path," 489.
55 The action plan focusing on the journey has been termed "implementation intention" and has been contrasted with "goal intentions," which refer to the general decision to achieve a goal; see e.g. Gollwitzer, "Implementation Intentions," 493.
56 See e.g. Knäuper et al., "Using Mental Imagery to Enhance Implementation Intentions."
57 Taylor et al., "Harnessing the Imagination."
58 See e.g. Dörnyei et al., *Motivational Currents*, 51–52. A good illustration is a church refurbishment project described by Malphurs (*Developing a Vision*, 162) in which the

chunks" not only makes the project more tangible and palatable, but it makes it also easier for everybody to find an area where they can meaningfully fit in and contribute. A key element in the success of the Vineyard movement has been John Wimber's insistence on "equipping the saints for the work of ministry" (Eph 4:12) so that, as he famously insisted, "Everybody gets to play"[59] – a route map of tasks made up of bite-size chunks can mobilise people effectively in this manner.[60]

Recruiting vision partners

The final strategy to be mentioned regarding the cultivation of vision is probably the most obvious one on the surface but one that is surprisingly hard to achieve in actual reality: *recruiting help*. The biblical description of God's dealing with Moses provides the classic illustration of this point, as the strategy was used with Moses not once but twice: first, after Moses complained about his inadequacy as a speaker to convey God's message to Pharaoh, God assigned Moses's brother, Aaron, "to serve as a mouth" for him (Exod 4:16); then, after Moses's bitter outcry of frustration about his inability to cope with fulfilling the divine vision for the Israelites (discussed earlier), God appointed 70 Elders to "bear the burden of the people along with you so that you will not bear it all by yourself" (Num 11:17). The Apostle Paul also had several helpers for his work, which becomes particularly clear when at the end of his ministry he suffered setbacks in this respect, and in 2 Timothy 1:15 he laments that "everyone in the province of Asia has deserted me." Clearly, he found it difficult to function well without assistants, as shown by the fact that in the final section of his letter he returns to the subject once again and tells Timothy, "Do your best to come to me soon, for Demas, in love with this present world, has deserted me and gone to Thessalonica; Crescens has gone to Galatia, Titus to Dalmatia. Only Luke is with me" (2 Tim 4:9–11).

We saw in Chapter 6 that the most effective visions for church communities tend to be *collective* in nature, with the "master-vision" accommodating the participants' individual dreams. Such a merger of personal and organisational dreams can result in a whole that is larger than the sum of its parts, which accentuates the need for consciously recruiting *vision partners* as an effective strategy to cultivate an initial vision. Maxwell reports that when he served as a church leader, he always tried to follow this principle

---

satisfaction of achieving one bite-size task led to taking on and accomplishing the next one, thereby starting an upward vision-spiral.

59 See Wimber, *Everyone Gets to Play*.

60 In a similar vein, Warren ("7 Ways to Help") advises church leaders that "As a part of vision-casting, you need to help individuals in your church see what they can do. Everybody will need to play his or her part in realizing the vision of the church. You'll need to give your congregation practical and immediate parts they can play in the process."

by engaging the whole leadership in developing and moulding his initial vision, also inviting several other church members with marked spheres of influence; as a result, he recounts, "By the time I went to the pulpit, the vision was never on the same level as when God first gave it to me; it was clearer and bigger. It was better because the body of Christ complemented what God had given me."[61] David Schmidt goes as far as to say that vision can *only* take on energy if it is shared; a collective flow of energy will build up as people feel that they have something valuable to contribute to the vision, as they are personally invited to embrace it, and as they hear their peers endorse it – this is, according to Schmidt, the key to the vision being adopted by a congregation.[62]

We should note, however, that despite the indisputable benefits of a vision that has been collectively shaped, Kouzes and Posner have observed that "All too often, leaders have come to assume that it is solely their responsibility to be the visionaries."[63] This, Kouzes and Posner warn, is not what the participants expect: "People don't really want to picture only the *leader's* vision. . . . They want to view themselves in the picture of the future that the leader is painting."[64] The profound maxim, "People support what they help to create" (already cited twice) is all too relevant here: people will become more effective if they are elevated from being vision executors to vision *partners*, and this "promotion" will not only strengthen them individually but will also bolster the collective vision itself.

Summary

The discerning of a divine vision, as discussed in the previous chapter, is an important step towards aligning one's life with God's calling, but it is only the first step in a longer process. This chapter began with the argument that the human capacity to behold vision has inherent limitations, and therefore in order that a vision be fully "complete," it will need to be actively cultivated by means of consciously strengthening and sustaining it. Vision has a tendency to "leak," that is, to lose some of its intensity and direction during the process of implementation. This is not entirely unexpected given that a God-ordained vision usually involves tasks that stretch the participants well beyond the limits of their perceived capabilities, which may make its accomplishment seem unattainable. This will inevitably result in some motivational "low points" during the realisation of a vision-inspired project, characterised by fatigue and discouragement, and this chapter has shown that even some of the main visionary figures in the Bible were no exception to this rule. And yet, people like Moses, Nehemiah and Paul managed

61 Maxwell and McManus, "Turning Vision Into Reality."
62 Schmidt, "Vision."
63 Kouzes and Posner, *The Leadership Challenge*, 107.
64 Ibid.

somehow to "run with perseverance the race set before them," indicating that it is possible to overcome the corroding effects of the various difficulties that are bound to come the visionary's way.

Proverbs 21:31 declares that "The horse is made ready for the day of battle, but the victory belongs to the LORD" (21:31), and while the second part of the proverb should be a source of comfort and confidence for believers, one needs also to bear in mind the first part, that is, the need to contribute to the victory by becoming "ready for the day of battle." Lessons drawn from the lives of biblical heroes as well as from research findings concerning the enhancement of mental imagery in psychology suggest several useful techniques to cultivate a Christian vision in the current age. The main themes of the strategies presented in this chapter concerned:

- Gaining strength, building confidence and overcoming fear through faith and trust in God.
- Enhancing the vision through sharpening the imagery, reactivating the vision regularly, bearing in mind the alternative outcome and celebrating progress and success.
- Dealing with obstacles through not being put off by criticism, exercising self-control, deriving inspiration from the perseverance of role models and learning from setbacks.
- Envisaging and fine-tuning a concrete roadmap to implement the vision, and breaking down the project into bite-sized tasks.
- Soliciting support from vision partners.

These techniques all have the capacity to nurture and reinforce a vision during the often challenging reality of everyday Christian living, and they can help to sustain its momentum until the final goal has been accomplished.

References

Augustine of Hippo. 2008. *Confessions*. Translated by Henry Chadwick. Oxford: Oxford University Press, 400.

Bandura, A. 1977. *Social Learning Theory*. Englewood Cliffs, NJ: Prentice-Hall.

Barna, George. 2009. *The Power of Vision: Discover and Apply God's Plan for Your Life and Ministry*. Ventura, CA: Regal.

Barnett, Tommy. 2005. *Reaching Your Dreams: 7 Steps for Turning Dreams into Reality*. Lake Mary, FL: Charisma House.

Best, Ernest. 1987. *Second Corinthians*. Interpretation. Louisville, KY: John Knox.

Betz, Hans Dieter. 1979. *Galatians: A Commentary on Paul's Letter to the Churches in Galatia*. Philadelphia: Fortress.

Brown, Raymond E. 1998. *The Message of Nehemiah: God's Servant in a Time of Change*. The Bible Speaks Today. Nottingham: Inter-Varsity Press.

Dillard, Raymond B. 1987. *2 Chronicles*. Word Biblical Commentary 16. Dallas, TX: Word Books.

Dörnyei, Zoltán. 2018. *Progressive Creation and Humanity's Struggles in the Bible: A Canonical Narrative Interpretation*. Eugene, OR: Pickwick.

Dörnyei, Zoltán, Alastair Henry, and Christine Muir. 2016. *Motivational Currents in Language Learning: Frameworks for Focused Interventions*. New York: Routledge.

Dörnyei, Zoltán, and Maggie Kubanyiova. 2014. *Motivating Learners, Motivating Teachers: Building Vision in the Language Classroom*. Cambridge: Cambridge University Press.

Dörnyei, Zoltán, and Ema Ushioda. 2011. *Teaching and Researching Motivation*. 2nd ed. Harlow: Longman.

Duncan, Rick. 2014. "Leadership Thoughts on Casting Vision." In *rickduncanlive. com*. http://cuyahogavalleychurch.blogspot.com/2014/09/leadership-thoughts-on-casting-vision.html.

Gollwitzer, Peter M. 1999. "Implementation Intentions: Strong Effects of Simple Plans." *American Psychologist* 54, no. 7: 493–503.

Gordon, V. R. 1988. "Self-Control." In *The International Standard Bible Encyclopedia, Revised*, edited by Geoffrey W. Bromiley, 386. Grand Rapids, MI: Eerdmans.

Guthrie, George H. 2015. *2 Corinthians*. Grand Rapids, MI: Baker Academic.

Harris, Murray J. 2005. *The Second Epistle to the Corinthians: A Commentary on the Greek Text*. Grand Rapids, MI: Eerdmans.

Henry, Alastair. 2015. "The Dynamics of Possible Selves." In *Motivational Dynamics in Language Learning*, edited by Zoltán Dörnyei, P. D MacIntyre and A. Henry, 83–94. Bristol: Multilingual Matters.

Hybels, Bill. 2002. *Courageous Leadership*. Grand Rapids, MI: Zondervan.

Hybels, Bill. 2008. *Axiom: Powerful Leadership Proverbs*. Grand Rapids, MI: Zondervan.

Knäuper, Bärbel, Michelle Roseman, Philip J. Johnson, and Lillian H. Krantz. 2009. "Using Mental Imagery to Enhance the Effectiveness of Implementation Intentions." *Current Psychology* 28: 181–86.

Kouzes, James M., and Barry Z. Posner. 2004. "The Five Practices of Exemplary Leadership." In *Christian Reflections on the Leadership Challenge*, edited by James M. Kouzes and Barry Z. Posner, 7–38. San Francisco: Jossey-Bass.

Kouzes, James M., and Barry Z. Posner. 2017. *The Leadership Challenge: How to Make Extraordinary Things Happen in Organisations*. 6th ed. Hoboken, NJ: Wiley.

Levering, Matthew. 2007. *Ezra and Nehemiah*. Brazos Theological Commentary on the Bible. Grand Rapids, MI: Brazos.

Longenecker, R. N. 1998. *Galatians*. Dallas, Tex: Word Books.

Lovejoy, Shawn. 2016. *Be Mean About the Vision: Preserving and Protecting What Matters*. Nashville, TN: Thomas Nelson.

Malphurs, Aubrey. 2015. *Developing a Vision for Ministry*. 3rd ed. Grand Rapids, MI: Baker Books.

Malphurs, Aubrey, and Gordon E. Penfold. 2014. *Re:Vision: The Key to Transforming Your Church*. Grand Rapids, MI: Baker Books.

Markus, Hazel, and Elissa Wurf. 1987. "The Dynamic Self-Concept: A Social Psychological Perspective." *Annual Review of Psychology* 38: 299–337.

Maxwell, John C. 2007. *The 21 Irrefutable Laws of Leadership: Follow Them and People Will Follow You*. Nashville, TN: Thomas Nelson.

Maxwell, John C. 2011. *Put Your Dream to the Test: 10 Questions to Help You See It and Seize It*. Nashville, TN: Thomas Nelson.

Maxwell, John C., and Ron F. McManus. 2000. "Turning Vision into Reality." *Enrichment Journal (on-line)* 5, no. 1.

McAllister-Wilson, David. 2004. "Reflections on Inspire a Shared Vision." In *Christian Reflections on the Leadership Challenge*, edited by James M. Kouzes and Barry Z. Posner, 55–68. San Francisco: Jossey-Bass.

Munroe, Myles. 2003. *The Principles and Power of Vision: Keys to Achieving Personal and Corporate Destiny*. New Kensington, PA: Whitaker House.

Myers, Jacob M. 1965. *Ezra, Nehemiah*. Anchor Yale Bible 17. New Haven, CT: Yale University Press.

Oyserman, Daphna, Elizabeth Johnson, and Leah James. 2011. "Seeing the Destination but Not the Path: Effects of Socioeconomic Disadvantage on School-Focused Possible Self Content and Linked Behavioral Strategies." *Self and Identity* 10, no. 4.

Rahner, Karl. 1967. *Spiritual Exercises*. Translated by Kenneth Baker. London: Sheed and Ward.

Schmidt, J. David. 2000. "So You've Got a Vision – Now What?". *Enrichment Journal (on-line)* 5, no. 1.

Stanley, Andy. 1999. *Visioneering: God's Blueprint for Developing and Maintaining Vision*. Colorado Springs, CO: Multnomah Books.

Stanley, Andy. 2004. "Vision Leaks." *Christianity Today/Leadership Journal*, Winter, www.christianitytoday.com/pastors/2004/winter/andy-stanley-vision-leaks.html.

Stanley, Andy. 2007. *Making Vision Stick*. Grand Rapids, MI: Zondervan.

Taylor, Shelley E., Lien B. Pham, Inna D. Rivkin, and David A. Armor. 1998. "Harnessing the Imagination: Mental Simulation, Self-Regulation, and Coping." *American Psychologist* 53, no. 4: 429–39.

Vohs, Kathleen D., and Roy F. Baumeister, eds. 2011. *Handbook of Self-Regulation: Research, Theory, and Applications* 2nd ed. New York: Guilford Press.

Warren, Rick. 2011. "Rick Warren's Challenge to the SBC Pastors' Conference." In *Pastors.com*. https://pastors.com/rick-warrens-challenge-to-the-sbc-pastors-conference/.

Warren, Rick. 2012. "7 Ways to Help Others Understand the Vision." In *Pastors.com*. https://pastors.com/how-to-share-gods-vision-for-your-church/.

Warren, Rick. 2018. "6 Ways to Prevent Vision Drift in Your Church." In *Pastors.com*. https://pastors.com/6-ways-to-prevent-vision-drift-in-your-church/.

Warren, Rick. 2018. "How to Start Growing toward Your Vision This Year." In *Pastors.com*. https://pastors.com/how-to-start-growing-toward-your-vision-this-year/.

Williamson, H. G. M. 1985. *Ezra, Nehemiah*. Word Biblical Commentary 16. Dallas, TX: Word Books.

Wimber, Christy, ed. 2008. *Everyone Gets to Play: John Wimber's Teachings and Writings on Life Together in Christ*. Boise, ID: Ampelon.

Conclusion
Becoming a "visionary" Christian

The first Christian sermon recorded in the Bible (in Acts 2) – delivered by the Apostle Peter at Pentecost – began by highlighting the significance of vision and then directly linked it to the release of the Holy Spirit into the world to dwell in the hearts of the followers of Jesus. Accordingly, Christian believers are, by definition, "visionaries" in the sense that a visionary channel has been activated in them to receive divine communication. This is consistent with Moses's yearning that everybody should be a prophet (Num 11:29) and Paul's placing of prophecy as the most highly valued spiritual gift (1 Cor 14:1). Having said that, the current book has not presented the archetype of a "visionary Christian" as a contemporary prophet (or mystic). In fact, very little of the previous discussion has concerned people with unique prophetic gifting, precisely because this gifting is seen as unique: while the Bible makes it clear that people do have different endowments, the faculty of vision was opened up at Pentecost to *every* disciple, potentially enabling *every* Christian to tune into the Spirit-empowered visionary wavelength that is serviced by the built-in faculty of mental imagery. It is this *generic* visionary capacity that has been the subject of this book, and seen from this perspective, a "visionary Christian" can be defined as anyone who utilises his/her inherent skills to receive and behold divine vision to good effect.

The main drive behind writing this book has been the recognition that in most, if not all, believers the visionary channel may not be functioning to full capacity. Although just as we know and prophesy only in part (1 Cor 13:9), we can also receive and behold vision only in part, the message of Scripture in this respect is not that we should patiently accept these limitations but just the opposite: 1 Corinthians 14:1 explicitly urges believers to "*strive* for the spiritual gifts, and especially that you may prophesy" (emphasis added). The understanding of this directive for the current work has been that while Christians may never be able to achieve perfect "spiritual communication skills" in their human lifetime, their competence in this area *can* be improved – or else why would they be encouraged to "strive" for it? Accordingly, this book has surveyed our existing knowledge about vision and mental imagery across a wide range of domains, from neuroscience and sport psychology to Ignatian spirituality and Christian leadership, with the stated purpose of offering tools for activating the visionary channel as much as possible. It was shown that this activation can happen at various levels, focusing on different facets of the visionary process.

Why is it important to improve the operation of the faculty of vision? This book has taken the position that the ultimate benefit of enhanced visionary skills is that they will allow people to align themselves better with God's specific purposes for them. That is, practising as a "visionary Christian" will help believers to find some answers to the age-old question in Matthew 19:16: "Teacher, what good deed must I do to have eternal life?" The specific answer will differ for each person, reflecting the fact that God has created everyone to have a unique role to play in the universe. This being the case, a book such as the current one can only hope to offer some building blocks for the foundation of such an enterprise. And yet, the overall lesson emerging from the previous discussions offers hope: through a combination of adopting a faithful, patient and prayerful disposition and drawing on one's innate faculty of vision, it may be possible to discern the special purposes that God has for humans.

Because the faculty of vision was activated at Pentecost in every follower of Christ, it needs to be reiterated that the skill of receiving and beholding vision is not restricted to prophets or church leaders only. The indwelling Holy Spirit enables every believer to receive divine communication through mental imagery in one way or another, sometimes in vivid picture sequences or dreams, and at other times through impressions of colours, sounds, feelings or intuitions, validated by an experience of joy, peace or the still small voice of the Good Shepherd. Although one does not have to be a leader to receive vision, one can certainly be made a leader through receiving vision; for example, his vision turned an African American clergyman born in segregated Georgia – Martin Luther King Jr. – into a prominent leader of the US civil rights movement and the winner of the Nobel Peace Prize for combating racial inequality. In his case, we are fortunate to have received a direct glimpse into his vision through one of the best-known vision statements of all time, the "I Have a Dream" speech.

This speech, delivered on August 28, 1963, is freely available to watch on the Internet,[1] and many will have heard at least some of the famous statements initiated by "I have a dream. . . ." What is particularly fascinating about these statements is that they were not scripted. Watching the whole speech, some may be surprised by how "normal" and "speech-like" the first part was, read out from sheets of paper to an audience of about 250,000 at a rather measured pace. At around the halfway point of the speech, however, Mahalia Jackson unexpectedly called out, "Tell 'em about the dream, Martin!" and it was as if an electric switch had been turned on: Rev. King

---

1 See e.g. www.youtube.com/watch?v=I47Y6VHc3Ms and www.youtube.com/watch?v=vP4iY1TtS3s.

put aside his prepared text, changed gear in his pace, pitch and emotion, and finished by describing an extended vision of a brighter future, punctuated eight times by the now legendary phrase, "I have a dream. . . ." Watching his delivery of these visionary lines, one can have little doubt that he had connected to some inner power that was not there a minute before – he had tuned into divine vision! The outcome of this connection was a vision statement that people still talk about some 55 years later.

There is a plaque outside Room 306 of the Lorraine Motel in Memphis, Tennessee, where the Rev. King was assassinated on April 4, 1968, with a quote from Genesis 37:19–20: "They said one to another, behold, here cometh the dreamer. . . . Let us slay him. . . . And we shall see what will become of his dream." The power of this dreamer's vision has been evidenced by history.

Author index

For Product Safety Concerns and Information please contact our EU
representative GPSR@taylorandfrancis.com
Taylor & Francis Verlag GmbH, Kaufingerstraße 24, 80331 München, Germany

www.ingramcontent.com/pod-product-compliance
Ingram Content Group UK Ltd.
Pitfield, Milton Keynes, MK11 3LW, UK
UKHW021440080625
459435UK00011B/323